Health Essentials

Herbal Medicine

Vicki Pitman (BA, MA–T, Dip HM), a native of South
Carolina, USA is a qualified herbalist, natural therapist,
teacher and writer. A member of The American Herbalists
Guild and tutor with the East-West College of Herbalism
in the UK, she also teaches introductory courses on herbal
medicine for the public. She conducts her practice, and lives
with her husband and three daughters, in Somerset.

The Health Essentials Series

There is a growing number of people who find themselves attracted to holistic or alternative therapies and natural approaches to maintaining optimum health and vitality. The *Health Essentials* series is designed to help the newcomer by presenting high quality introductions to all the main complementary health subjects. Each book presents all the essential information on each therapy, explaining what it is, how it works and what it can do for the reader. Advice is also given, where possible, on how to begin using the therapy at home, together with comprehensive lists of courses and classes available worldwide.

The *Health Essentials* titles are all written by practising experts in their fields. Exceptionally clear and concise, each text is supported by attractive illustrations.

Series Medical Consultant
Dr John Cosh MD, FRCP

In the same series

Acupuncture by Peter Mole
Alexander Technique by Richard Brennan
Aromatherapy by Christine Wildwood
Ayurveda by Scott Gerson
Chi Kung by James MacRitchie
Colour Therapy by Pauline Wills
Flower Remedies by Christine Wildwood
Homeopathy by Peter Adams
Iridology by John and Sheelagh Colton
Kinesiology by Ann Holdway
Massage by Stewart Mitchell
Natural Beauty by Sidra Shaukat
Reflexology by Inge Dougans with Suzanne Ellis
Self-Hypnosis by Elaine Sheehan
Shiatsu by Elaine Liechti
Spiritual Healing by Jack Angelo
Vitamin Guide by Hasnain Walji

Health Essentials

HERBAL MEDICINE

The Use of Herbs for Health and Healing

VICKI PITMAN

ELEMENT

Shaftesbury, Dorset ● Boston, Massachusetts

Melbourne, Victoria

© Element Books Limited 1994
Text © Vicki Pitman 1994

First published in Great Britain in 1994 by
Element Books Limited
Shaftesbury, Dorset SP7 8BP

Published in the USA in 1994 by
Element Books Inc.
160 North Washington Street,
Boston, MA 02114

Published in Australia in 1994 by
Element Books and distributed by
Penguin Australia Limited,
487 Maroondah Highway, Ringwood,
Victoria 3134

Reissued 1998

Cover illustration by Sally Townsend
Cover Design by Max Fairbrother
Printed and bound in Great Britain by
Biddles Ltd, Guildford & King's Lynn.

British Library Cataloguing in Publication
Data available

Library of Congress Cataloging in Publication Data
Pitman, Vicki
Herbal Medicine the use of herbs for health and healing
Vicki Pitman
p. cm. – (The Health essentials series)
Includes index.
ISBN 1–85230–591–6 $9.95
1. Herbs–Therapeutic use. I. Title. II. Series
OMC66.H33P58 1994
815′.321–dc20 94–23421 CIP

ISBN 1–85230–591–6

Note from the Publisher

Any information given in any book in the *Health Essentials* series is not intended to be taken as a replacement for medical advice. Any person with a condition requiring medical attention should consult a qualified medical practitioner or suitable therapist.

Contents

Acknowledgements

I would like to thank and give my appreciation to the outstanding teachers who have guided and inspired me in my herbal studies: Farida Sharan, Michael and Lesley Tierra, Dr Vasant Lad.

I extend thanks to my herbalist and Ayurvedic colleague Anthony Deavin for his valuable help; to my students and clients in Somerset who are also my teachers; and to the technical staff at Yeovil College for their assistance.

I am particularly grateful to my husband and daughters for their patience and cooperation; to my brothers and sisters for their support; and to my mother, who instilled in me a love of the wild.

Foreword

There is a beautiful tale told by the Cherokee of how the Green People came to the aid of human beings.

> In the beginning of this world, all creatures could speak a common language, and respected and understood one another, taking only what they needed to live. Gradually however, humans began to abuse their place in the Great Life: they took more than they needed, lacked respect for fellow creatures, trampled on others carelessly. The other animals held councils to try to decide how to solve the problem of man, but could think of no plan that would work. Finally the insects thought up the idea of giving diseases to humans to kill them off, and diseases began to appear among humans, but although many died, many survived. The insects then went to the Green People, the plants, for help in totally destroying arrogant humanity. After four days of deliberation, Grandfather Ginseng, the chief of the Green People, replied, 'We have heard your words and there is much truth in them. People have hurt and abused us as much or more than they have you. But we also understand that man is still young and foolish and we are all part of the same Great Life. So we have decided that if people come to us in a good way, a sacred way, we will help them by giving them the cure for every disease which you, the insects, have made.'

Based on a story related by David Winston, herbalist, Cherokee nation, in *American Herbalism*, Essays by Members of the American Herbalist Guild.

Introduction: Herbs for Healing

ERBAL MEDICINE IS humankind's oldest medicine and also the subject of much current scientific interest. It is as near to us as the geranium on the window-sill, the thyme in the garden, and the grass in the meadow. In using plants as medicines for health and healing we are acknowledging our place and our give-and-take relationship within the natural world. We are taking into our own hands responsibility for our health and well-being, and this naturally involves developing self-awareness and listening to our bodies. We are partaking of the harmony and vitality which our fellow beings have made available.

Plants have always been man's closest companions, for while we may survive without animals, we could not survive without plants. We tend to take plant life for granted yet it is our major source of food, shelter, clothing and fuels. Even the air we breathe is itself dependent on the activity of plants.

For all our scientific and technological skill, we cannot match that important plant process – photosynthesis – by which plant cells metabolize sunlight into energy for life and growth. Plants literally capture solar energy to help build their complex molecules of matter from soil minerals, oxygen and carbon which we in turn use as nutrients to give energy. In this exchange the light energy of the sun, through the mediation of plant life, becomes available to sustain human life.

Plants are our complementary partners in earth's ecology. As our lungs breathe in oxygen and give off carbon dioxide, plants take up carbon dioxide and release oxygen. As we use water and disperse it through the environment, plants take it up through

1

their roots. Their beauty of colour, shape, and fragrance augment the human experience, inspiring our thoughts and resonating with our deepest emotions. Just gazing on a plant or breathing its aroma can be deeply therapeutic. From ancient times our lives have been intertwined with those of our plant companions.

There is a saying among herbalists, 'Let your food be your medicine and your medicine be your food', a statement that recognizes there is no hard and fast division between a food and a medicine. Many common foods actually have therapeutic properties and can be used to heal; many plants we now consider only as medicinal herbs or even just as bothersome weeds have been part of the human diet for thousands of years. In addition our daily diet can be supplemented regularly with small quantities of herbs to actively maintain health and vigour and prevent disease – a practice common in many parts of the world. Herbs can be considered special foods that we turn to on a daily basis and in times of special need. Like best friends they are always there for us when we need them.

HERBAL MEDICINE

Herbal medicine, that branch of natural medicine that uses and values plants as potent allies in overcoming disease and maintaining health, makes use of the whole plant in treatments for the whole person. Like other natural medicine therapies, it views humans as part of nature and therefore observes and works with nature's gifts in the management of disease.

It is believed that within all of nature there exists a common life principle – the Vital or Life Force. This has been called *Chi* in Chinese, *Prana* in Indian and *Rooh* in Islamic–Tibb traditional medicine. The ancient Greeks knew it as *Pneuma*. The free flow and expression of this life principle, encompassing the mental, emotional and physical state of the person, constitutes health. Disease is said to result when this flow is obstructed or impaired, causing imbalances in the body which are experienced as the symptoms of illness.

Herbal medicine addresses itself equally to the 'terrain' or inner environment of the body within which the disease has developed and to the symptoms. Treatment with herbs is designed to resolve imbalances and restore the healthy function of the whole system, as well as particular organs. Plant energy can nourish and strengthen the whole body at the same time as it attends to particular symptoms. Herbs can treat the underlying, sometimes subtle causes of disease, as well as its manifestations as pain, inflammation or fatigue, and help to foster the positive natural healing force of the body. They can be said to work from the inside out as well as from the outside in.

Herbal medicine is an energetic medicine: it uses the qualities and energy of the herbs to influence and harmonize with the qualities and energy of the individual person, as the same life principle, or vital force, is common to both. Just as we recognize individual personalities by their characteristic behaviour, we can recognize individual herbs by their characteristic qualities and choose them to match the patterns of balance and imbalance in each person.

Herbal medicine is not an unscientific medicine, in using it we are not denying scientific knowledge or choosing superstition over fact. Every year more and more traditional remedies, once ridiculed by modern orthodox physicians, are being confirmed by scientific research and espoused by medical doctors as their efficacy is proven. Herbalists and other natural therapists are learning the scientific explanations for what they see happening in their clients.

The term 'natural' does not imply that whatever is straight from a plant is always and absolutely good and safe – any common food, even carrots, can become toxic when eaten in excess – but it does indicate that herbs can work with rather than override the body's natural healing activity, if they are used with knowledge, respect and common sense.

It is said herbal medicine uses the whole plant. This does not mean that all parts of the plant are always used, but that the part used – root, bark, leaves, flower or seed – will be taken complete as nature provided it. This contrasts with orthodox medicine which tries to isolate a single 'active' chemical component to give as medicine. Herbalists, while aware of these individual, prominent components of a plant, find that they work best when they stay with their natural molecular companions. This synergy – the combined effect of all the parts working together being greater than the sum of the parts working individually – helps keep herbal medicines free from damaging side-effects. With whole-plant medicine, one component affects one bodily part, while another component simultaneously affects a different part, both moderating each others' influences, balancing each other and creating a more balanced effect on the body.

Herbs and the Stages of Disease

Herbal medicine recognizes that the body has its own wisdom: inherently trying to stay healthy it chooses the best path available. The body deals with disease or imbalance by a distinct pattern of response ranging from acute, through sub-acute to chronic and degenerative.

Acute stage

The acute stage is an initial reaction phase to localize and eliminate pathogenic factors and excesses, and to recover from stress and trauma. In this stage the body's energy is strong and it may try to rebalance by creating a short-term, self-limiting crisis which is experienced as perhaps a cold, flu, earache, headache, skin eruptions or inflammation. Such things may sometimes be needed to force us to listen and pay attention to ourselves, to rest, or to adjust our diet. Although we call such experiences minor illnesses, they are the sign of a healthy body coping as best it can with the situation and signalling that things are out of balance, not right within. If we repeatedly ignore the signals, suppress the discomforts with drugs so we can carry on, without sorting out the underlying cause or imbalance, the disease may be driven deeper into the body and begin to affect more important organs. Antibiotics and other blocking drugs are strong medicines, very valuable in a life-threatening crisis, but the tendency to use them for every minor acute crisis is misguided because in suppressing the natural immune response they deplete the body's immune strength, leaving it weaker and actually contributing to imbalance.

Sub-acute stage

The sub-acute stage occurs when the body, by repeated efforts, has not successfully resolved its situation. Acute symptoms may have disappeared or appear only infrequently but the person will generally feel more tired and not quite right and lack zest for life. Here the body is containing the situation, using energy to compensate in various ways and may even continue for many years to maintain a 'balanced imbalance', but its immunity is gradually depleted and organ functions weakened.

Chronic stage

The chronic stage results if acute and sub-acute stages are not resolved; a more serious illness manifests itself and may become degenerative. The negative energy of the disease overcomes the positive efforts by the body. Organ functions become so weakened that the body cannot maintain itself properly.

Even in serious chronic diseases a person sometimes finds an unexpected source of healing energy and experiences a remission or cure. Such a source can be from the emotional or even spiritual dimension. It can also come from the energy of herbs. Herbalists recognize and try to work with these dynamics of the healing process, using herbs to support the body's efforts, clear the causes of disease and to be the catalysts for positive change.

The scope of this introductory book is that of the acute stages of short-term illness. If symptoms persist and in all other stages, please consult a qualified herbalist or medical doctor. For the minor upsets and symptoms of daily life, herbs are not only effective medicine, they help maintain the body's overall energy and strength, connect us to our wider environment, and enhance our self-awareness and the development of our intuitive nature.

1

The History of Herbal Medicine

THE ORIGINS OF herbal medicine date from the first human life, for humans have always used plants for food and medicine. The first herbals represent the recording of knowledge built up over millennia of experience and passed down through an oral tradition.

Knowledge about medicinal plants would have come from three main sources. Observation of animals and insects would have inspired many ideas for using plants as healers. Observing the characteristics of a plant and formulating ideas about its qualities, then trying it and experiencing its effects, would give knowledge. Similarly, carefully observing the effects of certain foods and flavourings and noting their particular qualities, would give ideas on how to use them in illness. Gradually through trial and error, aboriginal peoples came to know intimately the plants in their ecosystem. In some parts of the world, such peoples still exist and their knowledge is being tapped today, as pharmacologists looking for new drugs study the medicines of indigenous peoples.

Another way of gaining knowledge about plants, which is not scientific but which has been used by humans, is inner experience. In many cultures, certain persons have dreams or purposefully-induced altered states of consciousness in which they learn of the power of a particular herb for healing. In recent times, in the midst of western culture, the same process has created a unique method of herbal healing: the Flower Remedies of Dr Edward Bach. Such seers developed a form of direct perception of plants and their healing qualities.

In this small volume, it is only possible to trace the general outlines of the ideas and practices of herbal medicine based on written records, but it is important to remember that alongside this also runs the unwritten knowledge of the non-professional, mainly rural people – gathered, developed and passed from generation to generation and extant in every country – the so-called folk remedies.

Our earliest herbals date from about 3000 BC. Records from this period are found in India, where hymns of the *Rig Veda* are sung in praise of herbs; in China, where the *Yellow Emperor's Classic of Internal Medicine* details their use; and in Mesopotamia – the cradle of western culture – where Sumerian tablets record 1000 medicinal plants. It is interesting to note that several of these texts are actually religious documents, showing that knowledge of healing has always been part of an overall philosophical or spiritual tradition. This is certainly true of Chinese, Islamic-Tibb, and Ayurvedic medicine from India.

WESTERN HERBAL MEDICINE

Ancient Roots

Herbal medicine in western culture developed from its roots in Mesopotamia with particular contributions coming from Egyptian, Greek, Roman and Persian civilizations. Many herbs are also mentioned in Jewish writings.

In ancient Egypt, herbs were used for religious purposes, as cosmetics and for healing. Many plants, and even extraction methods, are depicted on the walls of tombs, indicating their central role in all aspects of life. Fragments of medical papyri from about 2000 BC give instructions and recipes for preparing various herbal medicaments including unguents, poultices and beverages made from herbs such as juniper, licorice, sweet calamus and aloe vera. Herbs were also extensively used in the mummification process.

The symbol we use today for prescription, ℞, derives from Egyptian pharmacists and is based on the single eye of the god Horus with an extending line and counter-stroke representing the spoon in which medicines were measured. The Greeks credit the Egyptians with starting the use of taking enemas for cleansing the body, a practice also used in Ayurvedic medicine.

The Greeks, great travellers and writers, were influenced by the waning Egyptian civilization, and incorporated in their practices some of its ideas – for example, that the starting point for all disease is poor digestion and elimination, leading to the circulation of toxic residues from the bowel into the body, a concept still central to naturopathy and herbal medicine, although now explicable in biochemical terms.

The medicine of Greece became the foundation of all later western medicine until the scientific revolution in the eighteenth century. The Greeks set up schools in the sense that men gathered in one place to learn from outstanding practitioners. They vigorously investigated the natural world and were as concerned to determine what actually constitutes and maintains health – much as other Greek thinkers explored the meaning of justice and beauty – as to describe and cure disease. The Greeks sought to establish the practice of medicine as a distinct craft, or *techne*, separate from both religious-based healing and folk medicine, though all three practices co-existed in their society. (It is striking how many herbs and plants find central roles in the Greek myths.) But Greek medicine was always practised within a comprehensive philosophical context.

Greek herbal healers

The Greek name most familiar to us today is probably that of Hippocrates, though it is now believed that writings attributed to him may actually be the work of several authors who were all associated with a famous school founded on the island of Cos around 430 BC by the first Hippocrates. These writings were developments of an earlier tradition of nature philosophers, or pre-Socratics, who pondered and formulated ideas about the nature of the cosmos and humanity's place in it. According to these philosophers all things derive from a primary substance, called *apeiron*, the unlimited, by Anaximander, or *pneuma*, spirit or air, by others. This substance is what gives life to matter and is found in every natural material. Thus man is a microcosm of the wider nature. There is also a life energy, *dynamis*, found materially in the elements of fire, earth, water and air which in turn form the bodily humours: phlegm, yellow bile, blood and black bile. In man, health and well-being depend on the right mingling, *krasis*, of the elements, establishing a state of *harmonia*.

In therapy, the Hippocratic writers applied what we would now term naturopathy or nature cure: the use of special diets, fasting, herbs and living according to a regime which harmonizes the particular balance of humours within each individual. The humoural concept was accepted in Greek society generally and influenced later philosophers. Plato evidently had high regard for physicians and their medical thought because he used them to explain his ideas about the nature of goodness and justice by comparing these to the ethics of medicine. In *The Phaedrus*, he describes the craft of the physician, and cites Hippocrates' belief that it is impossible to acquire medical knowledge about the nature of the body by looking only at its separate parts and without understanding it in its *holos*, or whole. Indeed our word holistic comes from the Greek *holos* as used in this context.

Two later Greeks also important in the history of herbal medicine were Dioscorides and Galen. Dioscorides, a surgeon in the Roman army, wrote a five volume *De materia medica* in the first century AD, which was subsequently used for centuries by herbalists. The one thousand entries were overwhelmingly herbs but also included animal and mineral substances. In the second century AD, Galen, a Greek physician in the employ of the Emperor Marcus Aurelius, praised Dioscorides' work and based much of his use of herbs on it.

Galen was a physician of considerable experience and wrote numerous treatises on the arts of medicine and on his investigations into anatomy and physiology, and also commentaries on the works of his predecessors and comtemporaries. From him we get an idea of the various practices and the debates going on between the physicians and schools of the time. His work contains the essence of the ancient Greek cosmology, its understanding of the nature of health and disease, and the concept of the four humours. He detailed their application to diagnosis and herbal therapy and there is evidence that he used the pulse as an indicator of the balance of the humours in his patients, much as Chinese acupuncture does. Because of his prestige and the survival of many of his writings, Galen was to be the dominant influence on all subsequent medical thought until the Renaissance, some sixteen hundred years later.

Islamic Medicine Grafted to the Greek Rootstock

With the end of the Roman Empire in the fifth century, communications and the exchange of ideas and practices in Europe became difficult. Knowledge fragmented and formal learning tended to stagnate during the next nine centuries. But when the eastern part was incorporated into the empire and civilization of Islam, which ran from North Africa into India, the medical learning of the Greeks and Romans was embraced by the Arabs. Its texts were preserved, studied, and used as a basis for their further development of medical knowledge and herbal remedies. Perhaps the most important Arab physician and teacher was the great Hakim, literally 'wise one' – Abu Ali al-Husayn Abd Allah Ibn Sina – known in the west as Avicenna.

Born in AD 980 Avicenna was a man of learning in many fields besides medicine – mathematics, astrology, and philosophy. He was widely travelled and renowned for his healing skills and was a court physician in Persia. He was an early chemist and perfected several processes such as filtration, sublimation, calcination and distillation – producing the first essential oil of rose. Avicenna wrote many books, the most famous being his *Canon of Medicine*, which greatly influenced the development of medicine and chemistry not only in the Middle East but also in Europe and India.

Arabian civilization established the practice of founding public hospitals and dispensaries for the sick. When the Moguls conquered parts of India, Arabic medicine went with them, where it both contributed to and learned from the Ayurvedic tradition. Today Arabic or Islamic medicine, known as Unani-Tibb, continues to be practised throughout its former empire, from north Africa to the Indian subcontinent and Indonesia. We in the West owe a great debt to this culture for its contributions to the healing arts.

Preservers of Herbal Knowledge in the West

Herbal medicine continued to be studied and used in Europe, by monks and nuns on the one hand, and by gifted individuals in a locality. The monasteries cared for their inhabitants and their visitors with herbs, maintaining special gardens for cultivating medicinal plants: when the Latin name of a herb includes the word '*officinalis*', it signifies that the plant was used by the monasteries. Among the people too, there was usually someone, often a wise woman, who had a knowledge of healing herbs. In the later Middle Ages and with the Renaissance in the fifteenth century, an explosion of learning began, stimulated by increased contacts with the Islamic empire through the Crusades. Ancient Latin and Greek texts were rediscovered and the first medical school was started in Salerno, Italy. The superior medical knowledge of the Arabs was eagerly sought, their texts re-translated into Latin and their teachers invited to teach in newly established medical schools.

A new broom sweeps clean

In the sixteenth century, the received medical wisdom was thoroughly jolted when a Swiss named Paracelsus began to question current practices which had tended to become corrupt and stagnant. Paracelsus saw physicians creating elaborate concoctions of dozens of exotic herbs and charging enormous fees, when he knew that in most instances simpler ones would have worked as well. For him, too, many exotic herbs were used and herbs in general used improperly because physicians merely practised without question what they had learned from text books and not from their own observations in the field. He came in like a new broom to sweep away the cobwebs.

Paracelsus was also interested in the new science of chemistry and the effect of metals on the human body, having seen new diseases appearing among local mine-workers heavily exposed to metals. He had his own laboratory and spent hours in investigations. But he remained equally devoted to the simple, local folk remedies, which he readily used. He gave them, however, a new guiding principle: discarding the humoural doctrine, he felt that each plant had a singular and specific action on specific diseases.

The age of herbal exploration

From the 1400s the newly consolidated European nation states such as Britain, France and Spain began their years of exploration and colonization of other parts of the world and it is fascinating to note that this major historical trend was in great measure prompted by the desire to secure the trade in herbs directly from India. At the time, herbs of the East were among the most sought after and expensive commodities of trade, not only for use in foods and perfumes but also for medicines, and the Arabs were the middlemen. It was while exploring a direct route to India that Columbus 'discovered' the Americas. In the wake of this and also new trade contacts with India and China, an explosion of interest in and collection of medicinal plants began. Specimens were brought back to be grown and their uses studied at such places as the Chelsea Physic Garden in London.

The traffic was not totally one way. In America, colonists brought with them their own herbs and, unintentionally, their own weeds hitching a ride as seeds embedded in clothing or among animals. Native American Indians were quick to make use of the medicinal ones such as plantain which they called 'white man's foot'.

In China the discovery of a new variety of ginseng from North America was welcomed and its curative properties so highly valued that a thriving trade began which continues to this day.

In the sixteenth and seventeenth centuries, new herbals began to be written, not in Latin for scholars and professionals, but in national languages, for an increasingly literate public. They incorporated contemporary experience and local herbs as well as the new herbs from foreign sources. One of the most famous of these was Nicholas Culpepper's *Complete Herbal and English Physician*. Culpepper intended it to be used by lay people, and as well as still using the humoural classification of herbs, he discussed them according to their astrological significance, for astrology was enjoying a revival at the time.

Parting of the Ways

During the next three centuries western medicine began to diverge from its common path with traditional herb-based systems. Physicians were becoming more and more influenced by the new developments in physics and chemistry. So much new knowledge – that now empowered humans with previously inconceivable mastery over natural forces – was being gained and so fast that gradually the general cultural outlook became one in which humans felt capable of eventually conquering every problem, including diseases, by manipulation of nature with the aid of technology. Instead of the universe consisting of elements of fire, water, earth and air, it was understood in terms of atoms and molecules. The idea of the balance and harmony between things changed to one of physical forces acting on matter in an exclusively material universe. The heart, for example, came to be seen in mechanistic terms as simply a pump, purged of its poetical-spiritual significance for health. The laws of physics and the discoveries of chemists now allowed matter to be manipulated. The individual constituents of herbs were capable of being isolated and analyzed as single entities, like the simpler compounds of metals. The word 'element' took on a new meaning denoting substances such as iron, gold or radium defined by their atomic weight, determined by the number of identical protons in their atoms. Herbs were gradually discredited as healers in favour of synthetic drugs.

Pasteur's perception of bacteria through the microscope shifted the whole thrust of medical science firmly away from sustaining health to heroically overcoming disease by the use of drugs to kill germs. The 'magic bullets' of vaccines and drugs did seem indeed to be capable of conquering disease altogether, and the scientists and doctors who delivered them soon became like gods or priests. The new medicines were credited with overcoming many dreaded diseases such as scarlet fever, diphtheria, and tuberculosis, though sanitation and improved living conditions played just as great a part in their demise. This trend has continued and accelerated in the twentieth century.

Root doctors to medical herbalists

Meanwhile, herbal medicine, though out of favour with the academic and scientific establishment, was not totally abandoned. The poorer, agricultural and working classes continued to depend on herbal remedies. In late eighteenth and early nineteenth century America, Samuel Thompson created a new system of herbal and naturopathic medicine based on the Indian use of herbs, especially the Indian tobacco, lobelia, and their methods of sweating and purging combined with his own research and experience. His method was to restore the 'vital heat' of the body with warming and stimulating herbs. Although he was hounded by the establishment who sought to prosecute him for murder, he was acquitted and his system became very popular because it worked, successfully curing yellow fever and other diseases. He eventually began to train agents to spread the practice of the system which he patented with the US government. One of his students, a Dr Coffin, brought his methods to England in 1838 where, as in America, they struck a chord with many people.

Another American and medical doctor, Wooster Beach, tried to steer medicine back to the use of herbs, and created a system called Eclecticism. He was ostracized by medical colleagues but again his methods were popular because they worked well. In both Britain and America these 'irregular' herbal systems existed alongside a growing medical science, professionals were trained, and hospitals were established and flourished. They were successful in curing hundreds of cases during the cholera epidemics. While often at odds with each other, they did have a common regard for the use of botanicals and the healing power of nature.

These 'irregular' botanic physicians, as they came to be known, were handicapped however, because by and large they did not belong to the educated classes and could therefore not command their respect – or access to funds. More and more funds were gradually put into establishing medical schools based on the laboratory-based science and their results received the prestige and publicity.

In Britain the herbalists just about hung on because their right to practise was protected by a charter from Henry VIII. They formed the Association of Medical Herbalists, (now the National Institute of Medical Herbalists) and in 1911 they founded a training school which continues to this day, having weathered many crises.

In the 1960s the outstanding herbalist Fred Fletcher-Hyde, with the help of thousands of ordinary users of herbal medicine who mounted a letter campaign, succeeded in establishing the right of qualified herbalists to practise and prescribe in their own right. This was included in The Medicines Act of 1968.

In America, the story is not so heartening. In the early part of the century a systematic campaign was launched by the American Medical Association to drive out the Irregulars altogether and make their practices illegal, even when people wanted to consult them. Herbal medicine was relegated exclusively again to the realms of folk medicine, and knowledge was kept alive largely by rural individuals, and by at least some Native Americans.

Continental contributions

On the Continent, while Pasteur's ideas may have captured the minds of scientists, the ideas of his friend and colleague, Claude Bernard, remained in the minds of some of the physicians and healers. Bernard had always insisted to Pasteur that while he conceded the existence of the bacteria, it was still more important, for healing diseases, to look to the 'terrain' in which the germs managed to survive. It was the condition of the 'terrain' or inner environment of the body which either allowed or prevented the germs causing a disease. In one sense the disease is seen as as the cure because it was what the body was doing to solve an untenable situation, an idea originating with Hippocrates.

Natural healers on the Continent like Father Sebastian Kniepp in the nineteenth century and later Dr Bircher-Brenner and Dr Vogel in the twentieth, continued to use herbal remedies in their successful cures. In France the traditional herbalist Maurice Messegué, though persecuted by the medical establishment, was justly famous and consulted by all manner of folk, including statesmen and celebrities. In Russia and Germany scientific 'progress' did not lead to such a rift between herbal and allopathic medicine and investigation of the efficacy of traditional herbs has meant that herbs are well respected in these countries and prescribed by doctors as well as by herbalists.

A Strong New Branch Sprouts in America

In America, one figure in particular stands out in the recent history of herbal medicine – Dr John Christopher who died in 1983. His life and work provide a link between the knowledge of the Irregulars and Eclectics, and the present day return of interest in herbal medicine. During the 1960s and 1970s many young people, having lost faith in allopathic medicine, went to learn from him and others like him. He became the godfather of a new generation of American herbalists.

Concurrently, native Americans, whose skills have always been a strong but unacknowledged part of American and European botanical medicine since the seventeenth century, began to share their traditions more openly with the now receptive white Americans. This development continues today.

Growth Renews in Europe

Similarly in Britain and on the Continent, in the past twenty years there has been a huge renewal of interest in practising herbal medicine as a career vocation. Older colleges find an increase in applications and newer ones have sprung up to satisfy the demand. Herbalists are continuing to improve their standards of training and increase public awareness of the safety and efficacy of herbal medicine.

HERBAL MEDICINE IN OTHER CULTURES

While herbalism has just about managed to survive in western culture and is growing again, it has never been abandoned by peoples and physicians of other cultures. Chinese medicine, in addition to its now well-known technique of acupuncture, also encompasses herbal medicine. Indeed the Chinese themselves feel that herbal and food therapy are the primary healing arts, the foundation of all others. The understanding of health and disease and methods of treatment have been developing continuously over about four thousand years. It rests on the concept of *chi*, energy, flowing as yin (the receptive female principle of the universe) and yang (the active male principle of the universe) in currents through the body, and on five elements interacting with each other. Today in China, though western medical diagnoses and treatments have been adopted, it has not been at the expense of traditional Chinese medicine which is still highly regarded. Practitioners of each will refer patients to the other. This is a situation greatly to be admired. In the west many herbalists are specializing in Chinese herbal medicine.

In India, *Ayurveda*, literally the science of life, has similarly survived the onslaught of western medicine, despite efforts to obliterate it during colonial occupation. It is now enjoying a higher status; colleges and hospitals train doctors in its methods and treatments. First written down in Sanskrit some two thousand years ago, Ayurveda has a distinguished history of healing, including highly advanced surgical techniques, herbal and food therapy, massage, rejuvenation techniques, gemstones and meditation, to ensure long and healthy life. Diagnoses and treatments are based on principles of *prana*-energy circulating in the body from the subtle regions and manifesting physically as the Five Elements and the Three Humours or *Tri Dosha: Vata, Pitta,* and *Kapha.* This tradition also is being successfully transplanted to the west.

From Native Americans we learn of another beautiful and profound understanding of natural medicine based on the Great Spirit and the Four Directions: North, South, East and West, each with their particular qualities of energy. These form the Medicine Wheel, within which we are born and journey as we evolve. Here again herbs play an integral part in the healing process and are valued as guides on this journey. Similar paradigms exist in other cultures.

THE FUTURE: FOOD FOR THOUGHT

Just as the old knowledge of the goodness of herbs for healing seemed destined to die out, it has been retrieved and is presently growing strongly. There is a new consciousness emerging with regard to herbal medicine. Pharmaceutical researchers are tremendously interested in investigating the properties of long over-looked herbs, such as turmeric, ginseng and even garlic. Ethno-botanists are contacting aboriginal peoples in Africa and South America who can tell them about the healing actions of local plants, and investigating practices which were once dismissed as mere pagan superstitions. Ironically, roles now seem to be reversed; the white man comes not as saviour but as supplicant. While much of the research is motivated by the old drive to find and isolate the magical 'active principle', it has at least caused scientists to respect herbal wisdom and to join with the environmentalists in calling for the saving of the earth's natural resources, including her plants and traditional peoples.

At the same time more and more people are using herbs and consulting herbalists. Consumers are demanding free access to them, and their voices are beginning to be listened to by government officials. While it is true that orthodox medicine has doubts about and sometimes feels threatened by herbal medicine, it is hoped that the continued efforts of the public and the practitioners together will eventually secure its status as a valuable, complementary part of national health care.

Today's herbalists embrace scientific research about herbs and their healing properties, finding that science most often turns out to validate the older knowledge, and they incorporate the results of scientific investigations of new plants into their practice. At the same time, herbalists are firmly rooted in their own traditions of natural medicine: healing comes from within; the whole plant is to be used; and the herbs are used to create the conditions in the body that allow the body's own intelligent, healing Vital Force to restore balance and health. Herbalists today are open to, even thirsting for, knowledge of herbs coming from the traditional medicines of China, India, Africa, the Americas and Australasia. There is a tremendous cross-fertilization of ideas taking place amongst herbalists and a global herbal wisdom is emerging.

2

How Herbs Heal

PLANTS ARE COMPLEX living entities. When they are used in healing, they are interacting with another complex living entity, the human body. The body breaks down the plant's identity and assimilates it into its own, and this process involves general as well as specific effects, three major areas of bodily function and several different levels of activity.

GENERAL AND SPECIFIC EFFECTS

When using whole herbs, healing is accomplished by a combination of multiple effects. A single herb can interact with several different aspects of the body simultaneously because of its complex energy and variety of biochemical constituents. The body has its own intelligence, or wisdom, and from among the different effects will take what it needs, eliminating the rest safely. Thus the overall effect of using herbs will be one of regulating bodily activity because they act to support homoeostasis, the body's regulating mechanism. So when used properly herbal medicine is very unlikely to seriously imbalance the body.

Herbalists consider this a tremendous advantage over drug therapy because while one constituent gives the plant a characteristic action, such as a diuretic one, others are simultaneously affecting other aspects of the body and serve to round out the main action. This multiple effect also means that several herbs

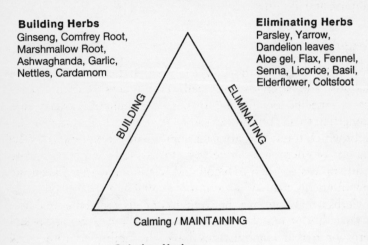

Building Herbs
Ginseng, Comfrey Root,
Marshmallow Root,
Ashwaghanda, Garlic,
Nettles, Cardamom

Eliminating Herbs
Parsley, Yarrow,
Dandelion leaves
Aloe gel, Flax, Fennel,
Senna, Licorice, Basil,
Elderflower, Coltsfoot

Calming / MAINTAINING

Calming Herbs
Chamomile, Scullcap, Valerian,
Lemon Balm, St. John's Wort, Hops

Figure 1   The Triad of Bodily Functions

may be used successfully for the same ailment, so our range of choice is very wide indeed. The specific therapeutic effects of herbs are described in Chapter Four.

The Triad of Bodily Functions

At any time the body is:

- Breaking down food and air and building new cells and tissues
- resting and recuperating and repairing
- eliminating waste by-products of metabolism and digestion.

These three bodily functions form a triad of balanced health, each side of which should be roughly equal to the other two. It is an active, dynamic balance – adjusting itself constantly in response to the changing inner and outer environment. If the building or the eliminating side becomes either deficient or too dominant, or there is not adequate rest and repair, the health of the person suffers. Herbs can be said to nourish, support or activate each of these three functions and herbalists describe them as tonifying, calming and eliminating.

Tonifying

Herbs can improve the body's ability to perform its task of building and strengthening cells and tissues. Certain herbs act on specific organs and tissues to stimulate, nourish and strengthen them and thus to 'tonify' their function. For example, herbs which tonify the stomach improve digestion, and thus the amount of energy we derive from food. Herbs which stimulate bodily processes, such as blood and lymph circulation, keep the flow of energy free and ensure it is available to every cell.

Herbs which improve the strength of cells overcome weakness or flaccidity of muscles, nerves and membranes. Some special herbs or herbal combinations have the ability to tonify the essential energy of the body and these are called Energy tonics. Ginseng is one such herb.

Calming

Complete relaxation allows the body to rest and repair, to return to a state of equilibrium, to recover from exertion. This is accomplished primarily through the parasympathetic nervous system (nerves leaving the lower end of the spinal cord connected with those in or near the soft internal organs) in concert with the hormones. Overstimulation or overwork of any organ, tissue or system, will eventually weaken function and insidiously undermine health. Even emotional upheavals may lead to stress and tension which can stay locked in the body. Herbs which support the nerves and endocrine glands allow the body to recuperate and renew its energy.

Eliminating

Elimination and internal cleansing is as important to health as building. The elimination and cleansing in the body is the responsibility of the kidneys, liver, lungs, skin, lymph and colon. If any one of these systems becomes overburdened by excess and cannot complete its cleansing functions, the body tissues gradually become toxic with the rubbish. Herbs have the ability to enhance the cleansing processes of the body: to break up congestion, neutralize toxins and to promote their elimination. Used in conjunction with good diet they will keep this important aspect of the health triad fully functioning.

In reality the bodily functions cannot be separated but overlap and are dependent on each other. For example, to provide proper elimination, the kidneys must be both in good tone and have periodic 'rest'; and a hyperactive nervous system can overstimulate metabolism generally. Herbs have the ability to support more than one of these aspects at the same time.

Regular use of herbs supports the body as it constantly maintains its healthy balance, but our plant companions are also there to assist us when imbalances lead to illness.

Herbal Activity

Herbs affect the body on several different levels simultaneously: the nutritional, biochemical, psycho-emotional, and energetic.

The nutritional level

Many herbs can be used as foods. Others can supply significant quantities of nutrients such as vitamins, minerals, and starches. These include lemons, dandelion roots and leaves, burdock roots, nettles and garlic. Herbs can actually be combined to give an excellent mineral and vitamin supplement. Valerian (*Valeriana officinalis*) for example, known for its relaxing effects on the nervous system, contains a high proportion of the mineral calcium needed by the body for healthy nerve function. Consuming herbs regularly in small amounts along with meals helps preserve health and prevent disease.

The bio-chemical level

Plants, whether medicinal herbs or foods, are complex chemical packages. For example, the potato contains over one hundred and fifty identified substances, as well as numerous others which remain unidentified. The same is true of medicinal herbs. While science has elucidated many of their most important active constituents, no doubt new ones will continue to be discovered. The

main active constituents often explain a herb's most characteristic action: tannins, for example, are responsible for astringent,
antiseptic and wound-healing actions; some glycosides have sedative, others purgative, effects. But understanding the activity of
herbs according to this paradigm is less useful than understanding
that a herb is a complex of many different compounds and it
is the known therapeutic effects of all these together – the
synergistic effect – which is the best guide to its use. (When
such active constituents are isolated and given medicinally, as
in drug therapy, the strength of their action increases, often
dramatically, creating unwanted or negative side-effects.)

The main medicinally active constituents are the tannins,
alkaloids, volatile oils, mucilages, acids, glycosides, and bitters.
Readers are referred to Further Reading in Chapter 8 for
additional information on these.

Psycho-emotional level

We have said that herbal medicine aims to treat the whole
person, including their mental and emotional aspects. In general
herbs which are cooling and/or heavy are used to ground, calm
and sedate. Those which are light and stimulating are used to
clear stagnation, to uplift and invigorate. For example, when
the fluid congestion and bloating that can accompany the
menstrual period is reduced, symptoms of irritability and anxiety
are relieved. Herbs which are sweet nourish, strengthen and
comfort. Aromatic herbs also affect the mental-emotional level
and play an important role in treatment of psycho-emotional
problems. Often when congestion and blockages at the physical level are cleared, through the appropriate herbal strategy,
mental-emotional clarity and peace are restored.

The energetic level

In a sense when we take herbs they are transferring to us the
harmonious flow of Vital Force which they have developed
in order to survive, and it is their energy that resolves the
disharmony in ourselves causing disease. The recognition of this
phenomenon is at the foundation of traditional medicine
systems – Tibb (Greek-Islamic), Chinese, Ayurvedic and
American Indian. It is important to note that although this

knowledge may be in one sense pre-scientific, it is not necessarily unscientific. It includes scientific understanding but also goes beyond it.

Energetic understanding of herbs is a holistic, comprehensive understanding because it takes into account all dimensions of a plant's nature not just the biochemical-physical. Understanding the energetics of herbs and how these harmonize the energetic pattern of the particular individual, enables us to create the most effective herbal preparations and heal at the deeper levels.

Energy Herbs

A recent development in the understanding of how herbs work has come from researches into what causes stress and the relationship between certain tonic herbs and the body's recovery from stress.

The Chinese have a special category of herbs called *Chi* or energy tonics which they have found to restore and rebuild the body's life energy, even when a person is near death. The most famous of these is ginseng. Scientific research on ginseng has provided some clues as to how it works. As Stephen Fulder reports in his book, *About Ginseng*, researchers have found ginseng to have unique and remarkable effects leading them to coin a new term for this class of herbs – 'adaptogens'. Adaptogens increase the body's ability to adapt to stress positively, indeed to survive extremely stressful situations. It is unclear exactly how this occurs, but the plant's action is believed to affect the hormones and nerves, and their response to the environment. In effect ginseng energizes the whole body.

It is possible that as well as single herbs, certain combinations of herbs may be created whose combined effect also affects energy directly. Several cultures seem to have a famous tonic which is believed to be an elixir of life. One such combination may be *Chayavan-prash*, a highly respected Ayurvedic formula, taken regularly to maintain overall health. As stress is recognized as being an important contributor to many chronic diseases, this new understanding of the abilities of herbs to revitalize is very welcome. As we open our minds and hearts to herbal healing, there may be many more uses yet to be discovered.

3

Herbal Energy and Constitutional Types

THE LIFE FORCE expresses itself on the physical level as different qualities or patterns of energy – much as a river has different characteristics and qualities of movement depending on whether it is flowing as a rushing mountain stream, a broader lowland river or a wide, silt-laden delta. This expression manifests as the phenomena of Earth, Water, Fire, Air, and Ether: substances ranging from the most solid to the most ethereal. These manifestations, or elements, are present in differing degrees and combinations in the human body, in plants and throughout nature.

It is significant that each of the major known traditional medical systems of the world developed independent but similar paradigms of energetic understanding to make sense of the natural world, health and disease. These may be described in slightly different terms and configurations of the patterns – perhaps reflecting differences of climate, geographical and cultural experience – but it is sensed that they are descriptions of the same phenomenon. In this book, the paradigm of Ayurvedic medicine is chosen as the model. It is very similar to our own European-Greek humoural tradition, includes many herbs in common, and has the advantage of still being actively and successfully practised today, after five thousand years.

THE ELEMENTS

The elements show different combinations of qualities such as dryness and moisture, heat and cold, lightness and heaviness, mobility and inertia. These are not present in absolute form, but are tendencies within a continuum and are relative to their opposites.

- **Earth** manifests the qualities of solidity, firmness, heaviness, density and cold
- **Water** manifests the qualities of heaviness, fluidity, cold and moisture
- **Fire** manifests yet more activity, also heat, light and colour, and less density
- **Air** manifests to a greater degree the qualities of mobility, lightness (less weight) and dryness, and tends to be colder.
- **Ether** manifests as emptiness, that positive space within which the other elements function, find their expression and communicate or interact with each other. Its qualities are clarity and subtlety. At the emotional-mental level it is the space which allows free expression of one's true nature. Spiritually it is the inner space, emptied of mental activity, wherein the individual consciousness becomes aware of the cosmic spirit. This is the most subtle manifestation of the Life Force.

Each of these elements is present to greater or lesser extents in all of nature from stones to sub-atomic particles. For example, in humans Earth would be the most obvious and most characteristic element of bones, teeth and to a lesser extent muscles because these are the most dense and solid tissues in the body. Water is present in great quantities in our bodies but is most obvious in mucous membranes, in the lubricating fluid around joints, in blood and in lymph fluid. Similarly, Fire is manifested in the digestive acids, in that veritable chemical factory, the liver, and in the warmth and redness of blood. Air is represented in the electrical impulses of the nervous system with its qualities of rapid communication and instigation of movement. Even Ether – space – is necessary in the body and is represented in, for example, the thoracic cavities, the colon, and the synaptic space through which nerve impulses are transmitted.

In herbs, the elemental energy is expressed in such things as the earthiness of bark and roots; the fluidity of sap; the fire of colour in flowers and the chemical process of photosynthesis; the breathing of air by leaves; and the space within which the seed forms and is carried.

HERBS AND THEIR ENERGETIC QUALITIES

Four main qualities characterize herbs: warmth, coolness, dryness, and moistness. These describe the energy effect herbs have in the body as cooling, warming, drying, or moistening, some herbs being more cooling or warming than others. Cayenne, for example, is much hotter than black pepper. In some herbs the degree of heat or coolness is so similar to that of the human body that it is considered neutral. Each herb will have its characteristic energy effect on the body according to the composition of the elements within it.

Warming herbs stimulate metabolism, adding heat, and stimulate the body's energy. But a very heating herb will also have a drying effect if used for long enough, and eventually a depleting effect if the body is overstimulated, so it is recommended more for short-term use in those with dry symptoms, Air imbalance, or weakness.

Cooling herbs counteract excess heat in the body – fevers or inflammations. They help the elimination or clearing of heat through the sweat glands, kidneys, liver or colon.

Moistening herbs, often barks or roots with a starchy, fibrous or soft texture, impart a demulcent, softening, soothing effect to dry, inflamed or irritated tissues and strengthen the basic fluid essence of the body, the Water humour.

Drying herbs are either astringent in effect – drying excess water in tissues by a tightening, binding action – or stimulating to the urinary and circulatory systems which increases the elimination of water via skin or the kidneys. They are good for excess damp conditions such as swellings and catarrh. Herbs can exhibit two qualities at the same time, though one may tend to be its primary effect.

Another way traditional herbal medicine has of recognizing these qualities is through taste and it is a guide to understanding the healing effect a herb will have. The bitter taste is strongly cooling, and stimulates detoxifying; the pungent taste strongly heating, drying and stimulating; the salty taste mildly warming, moistening and solidifying; the sour taste warming and drying; the sweet taste very warming, solidifying and moistening; and the astringent taste mildly cooling, drying and tonifying.

The energetic pattern of a herb is the key to knowing what its effect or action will be on an individual body. When this is matched to the energetic pattern of the person who is ill, the healing effect will be more accurate and successful.

THE THREE HUMOURS AND THE CONSTITUTIONAL TYPES

In the body the elements of Earth, Water, Fire, Air and Ether mingle to create three distinct patterns of energy, or 'humours' as they are called in Ayurvedic and Greek-Tibb medicine. (These correspond roughly to the concepts of Yin, Yang and Wind in Chinese medicine.) As all the elements are present in each of us, so are each of the humours, but in varying degrees. The predominant ones indicate our predispositions, our constitutional type or temperament.

The Three Humours

Earth and Water together constitute the Water humour (*kapha*). Fire combines with some degree of Water's fluidity to constitute the Fire humour (*pitta*). Air and Ether taken together constitute the Air humour (*vata*). Like the elements the humours are expressed in the body's anatomy and physiology; for example digestion and circulation relate primarily to the Fire humour, mucous and urine to the Water humour and nerves and movement to the Air humour. The humours also find expression at the more subtle level of emotional and mental make-up.

Constitutional Types

Some of us are born with a tendency to be strong in one humour, others perhaps in two and some may have a more even distribution of humours. We may be a Water-predominant type, a Fire type or an Air type; or perhaps a Water-Fire, Earth-Air or Fire-Air type. The characteristic temperament at birth may become modified, imbalanced or even obscured by life's experiences and activities such as emotional traumas, diet, exercise or lifestyle. Our particular mix of humours can also predispose us to certain types of illness when we become unbalanced. This is because the predominant humour will also be the one to most easily tip into excess and cause imbalance, though any of the humours can become imbalanced given a particular set of negative circumstances in our lives. Factors which often cause the humours to become out of balance include excessive stimulation, traumas and the accumulation or blockage of a particular humour by lifestyle, diet, exercise or environment.

Each humour can act as either a positive or negative factor in our lives depending on whether or not it is in balance with the other two and with our current environment – just as we need a certain amount of physical fire in our bodies for warmth but not so much as to dry out our tissues. Similarly, there may be times, when we need to become a little fiery in order to defend ourselves, both physiologically – the immune response of the body is a function of the fire energy – and emotionally. At other times we need to express love or find new ways of thinking and responding in order to change and develop – aspects of the Water and Air humours. The positive quality of each humour indicates the one to activate and support with herbs and food when restoring harmony.

The following is a brief description of the characteristics of the constitutional types.

We all have each of the humours within us and each will manifest more strongly at different stages of life or given enough imbalance. For simplicity's sake those constitutional types described here are only of one main humour dominance. Childhood and winter are typically the time of the Water humour; youth and adulthood, spring and summer are the time of the Fire humour; older age and autumn the time of the Air humour. Although Water types are more inclined to experience phlegm and mucous excess, over-exposure to cold and damp can imbalance the Water humour in other types too.

Fire type

A Fire-type person tends to be perceptive, goal-oriented, efficient and practical. She knows her own mind. On the physical level, she will have good digestive fire, warm circulation and a medium body-build. Of the three constitutions, the Fire type is the most prone to digestive problems such as acidity or heartburn, heavy menstrual periods, or skin complaints such as acne, as it is easiest for this type to become imbalanced by additional heat – whether mental, emotional, or physical. The Fire type is also most easily irritable, angry and will tend to overwork.

Herbs for Fire types or imbalanced Fire include cooling herbs or neutral herbs such as coriander, cumin, turmeric, borage, burdock, red clover, licorice, asparagus. Avoid too much heating, spicy herbs like chillies, and sour, fried and salty foods.

Water type

A Water-type person tends to be strong, steady and calm, compassionate, and placid. He may need financial security, and seems to attract it, and may be quite attached to loved ones. On the physical level, this type will be of heavier build and prone to overweight, water retention or respiratory congestion because with a predominance of Water it can more easily become excessive in these areas. Over-concern, stagnation, introversion, depression or rigidity of attitude are the negative aspects of the Water humour.

Herbs for Water types or imbalanced Water include warming, metabolic stimulants like cayenne, black pepper, thyme, rosemary, garlic, sage and eucalyptus; draining herbs like juniper, chickweed, cleavers and dandelion; dispersing herbs like basil and yarrow. Water types should avoid sweet and rich or processed foods and salt.

Air type

The Air-type person tends to be flexible in mind and body, especially sensitive to surroundings and to change, and quick to react to new things. The keynote for her is variation and irregularity. The Air type tends to a lighter frame, less substance and to feel cold, preferring warmth and light. She can be excited and intensely active, then tire and need rest. When imbalanced, physical symptoms may be those of stiffness, nervousness or hyperactivity, dryness or lack of energy and endurance. On the mental-emotional level, imbalance shows as indecisiveness, feelings of anxiety, insecurity or lack of confidence.

Herbs for Air types or imbalanced Air include grounding, relaxing or warming herbs like valerian, chamomile, catnip and ginger; tonic or moistening herbs like comfrey, dong quai (Chinese angelica), licorice, slippery elm, kelp, honey, fenugreek, oats and oatstraw.

Type assessment

Awareness of one's constitutional make-up leads to a greater understanding and acceptance of oneself and of others. We realize why a particular food – or even a person – upsets us: it is probably because it aggravates too much a particular humour or tendency in us. We can discern the best food, herb or activity that will restore that harmony of our particular blend of humours. The awareness gives positive guidance in how to minimize our limitations and make the most of our strengths by seeing them in the context of the overall dynamic flow of Energy in us. We have the means to avoid to a greater extent those conditions which lead to disease, or to resolve imbalances before they become an ailment – the means of taking responsibility for our health.

For this purpose use the Humour Assessment table on pages 32–4. Completing this form will enable you to know yourself, your strengths and weaknesses, and your tendencies when imbalance occurs. Herbs may then be chosen more accurately to restore or maintain your balance. Tick the column that best describes your overall tendency in each category throughout your life in general, not just most recently. You will find different aspects of yourself fall under each humour, which is normal. Total the number of ticks in each column; the results will give you a good idea of the strength of each humour in yourself. It is a good idea to photocopy the pages and repeat the assessment at intervals. As your self-awareness develops you may find you change your mind over one or more items, and proportions can be adjusted.

Table 1 Humour Assessment

	WATER (Earth and Water)	FIRE (Water and Fire)	AIR (Air and Ether)
Structure (Physique)	Sturdy. Large bones, chest. Tends to overweight	Medium build and weight.	Slender. Small bones, chest. Light or underweight.
Hair	Thick, abundant, often wavy. More body hair.	Oily, straight, blonde, red. Tends to baldness.	Fine, dark. Can be kinky (irregular).
Skin	Moist, soft, fair to pale, thick, cool.	Moist, oily. Tends to moles, freckles, birth marks, acne.	Patchy dry or rough, thin, dark, cold. Veins prominent
Appetite	Moderate, steady. Prefers sweet tasting foods.	Strong. Needs food to be content and to work.	Variable, but feels 'spacey' without food.
Digestion	Sluggish. Food 'sits' in stomach.	Efficient, fast. Tends to acidity.	Irregular, worse with change or travel.
Exercise and movement	Moves slowly or with reluctance, sedentary. Prefers slowness, conserves energy.	Active, prefers competitive sports.	Active but tends to restlessness or tossing, nervous movement.

	WATER (Earth and Water)	FIRE (Water and Fire)	AIR (Air and Ether)
Stamina and energy	Strong. Slower to start but steady. Good endurance.	Moderate. Focuses energy. Tends to overwork.	Low or fluctuating. Quick to start & to stop. Intense energy, then fatigue.
Stools	Moderately frequent, heavy with mucous. Tends to sluggishness.	Regular (one or more a day), large, soft, yellow-tinged.	Variable, affected by slight change (e.g. travel). Tends to dryness, hardness or constipation.
Sweat	Moderate.	Easily produced, profuse. Sensitive to heat.	Little, not easily provoked.
Urine	Moderate. Tends to milky colour.	Profuse. Can be red or burning when imbalanced.	Scanty, less colour.
Circulation and body temperature	Moderate to cool. Least sensitive to changes. Copes well with extremes (e.g. of heat and cold).	Strong, feels warm. Sensitive to heat.	Feels cold, and feels 'the cold.' Disturbed by uneven temperatures, changes, wind

	WATER *(Earth and Water)*	FIRE *(Water and Fire)*	AIR *(Air and Ether)*
Sleep	Sound. Enjoys long sleep. Slow to waken. Tends to excess.	Moderate, uninterrupted. Mind controls sleep, 'Night owl'.	Light. Easily disturbed, wakes early. Morning is best time.
Dreams	Romantic, emotional.	Colourful, involve conflict, passion.	Active. Involve movement e.g. flight, falling.
Mental, emotional and life style	Thinks slowly, carefully. Retains well. Good administrator. Compassionate, devoted, patient, calm, prudent, sentimental. Desires security (e.g. financial, love).	Sharp, penetrating, practical, articulate, knows own mind. Clarity of thought. Avid reader, likes to be busy, competitive, ambitious, judgemental. Teacher, leader	Open mind. Alert, quick to learn and to forget; to grasp & to reject. Talkative, active, tends to be restless and overly sensitive, enjoys travel and change. Flexible. Communicator.
Most likely negative emotion	Grief	Anger	Anxiety and fear
Areas of focus of imbalances	Respiratory, mucous. Congestion, inertia, water retention, weight gain.	Digestive, liver, skin. Fevers, inflammations. Irritability.	Insomnia, stiffness, nervous or mental distress.
Totals			

4

The Therapeutic Actions of Herbs

A NY HERB PRODUCES several of the therapeutic actions that may simultaneously affect the body and which are moderated by that body's energetic pattern. A knowledge of main actions described here combined with a knowledge of humoural constitution, or temperament, allows the reader to form a successful herbal strategy.

CARMINATIVE ACTION

Examples: cloves, ginger, cinnamon, coriander, cardamom, cumin, chamomile, fennel, dill, caraway, allspice, sweet calamus, cayenne pepper or paprika, asafoetida, fenugreek, rosemary, sage, thyme, marjoram, basil.
Caution: while safe for occasional teas, culinary and short-term use, in pregnancy avoid prolonged or concentrated use of cinnamon, sweet calamus, thyme, sage, rosemary, fennel, fenugreek and marjoram.

This action affects the digestion and assimilation of foods and the elimination of digestive residues such as gas. Carminatives are usually flavourful and include many of our common spices and seasonings. They are also effective medicines for digestive and intestinal symptoms.

In Water temperaments their digestive fire is liable to be low or sluggish and they benefit from the most warming carminatives such as ginger, pepper and garlic. In Fire types the tendency is for it to be a little too high so the mild carminatives, cumin and fennel, are helpful. In Air types, digestion and eating habits tend to be variable; they benefit most from warming and also sweet carminatives like ginger, cinnamon and cloves. (Digestive bitters, such as yellow gentian root, while not pleasantly flavourful like carminatives, stimulate the digestive enzymes, tonify the stomach, and thus improve overall health, especially in cases of ulcers or weakness and debility.)

The Importance of Digestion

Because of our prevailing lifestyle with its emphasis on fast, processed, convenience meals and almost constant stimulation, digestion in many people becomes weakened. If we eat while feeling strong emotions: grief, anger or irritability, depression or anxiety, we are in a sense eating these emotions along with the food and this too affects digestion.

Through the process of digestion the human body converts and assimilates the energy needed for life from food. Even the highest quality food, unless well prepared and then well digested, can lead to imbalances in the system and blockages in circulation of blood and nutrients. Carminatives improve and strengthen digestion and, if used on a daily basis, balance the overall energetic effect of foods on our bodies. A food with a cold energy such as cold milk, or cheese – which would be slightly imbalancing for a Water temperament, especially in winter – when combined with a warming carminative herb such as ginger, clove or cardamom and served warm becomes a more balanced food for that person and the herb-food combination a new synergistic entity.

LAXATIVE ACTION

Examples: slippery elm, senna, plantain (psyllium) seed, rosemary, licorice, turkey rhubarb, raspberry leaves, dandelion, ginger, black pepper, cayenne pepper.
Caution: while safe for occasional teas, culinary and short-term use, in pregnancy avoid prolonged or concentrated use of cayenne, senna or rosemary, and any use of turkey rhubarb. Avoid licorice in presence of water retention, oedema, hypertension, and cardio-vascular conditions. Senna should only be used for limited short terms.

This action regulates and balances good bowel elimination. Some of these herbs stimulate metabolism, some moisten and soften the contents, adding bulk, some tone the smooth muscles or stimulate the gall bladder to release bile, the body's natural laxative.

Ginger or cayenne would most benefit Water types; rosemary combined with slippery elm in milk would help Fire types; ginger with psyllium seed, flax seed or aloe vera gel work well for Air types. Raspberry and rosemary tonify the peristaltic muscles. If any cramping or griping effect is experienced when taking laxative herbs, combine them with warming antispasmodic herbs (see Nervine Action page 44).

The Importance of Colon Health

Next to good digestion and assimilation, good bowel elimination of waste and the by-products of metabolism is extremely important to maintaining or recovering good health. Bowels need to move regularly and easily at least once a day. Colon congestion can result from dietary, emotional and stress factors. If wastes are allowed to remain in the body for prolonged periods, the effect is the same as if we fail to empty our kitchen waste-bins regularly, producing the ideal environment for unwanted bacteria, viruses and yeast (*Candida*) to thrive. Bowel function can also both reflect and influence our emotional state. Tendencies to retain negative feelings – for example, self-doubt, uncertainty, anger or anxiety – without expressing or resolving them positively, can lead to a 'hanging on' in this aspect of our physical selves. Herbs can effectively cleanse and restore good bowel elimination, and a general sense of lightness, confidence and emotional well-being usually ensues.

BLOOD PURIFYING ACTION

Examples: turmeric, red clover, golden seal, marshmallow root, echinacea (cone flower), chaparral, burdock, yellow dock, St John's wort, garlic, thyme, honeysuckle.
Caution: while safe for occasional teas, culinary and short-term use, in pregnancy avoid prolonged or concentrated use of thyme and garlic; avoid golden seal altogether. Golden seal is best

restricted to short-term use generally. Chaparral is currently under review for possible toxicity and is best avoided.

This action – also called alterative, heat clearing and Fire reducing – clears excess heat in the blood and body. Excess heat may be caused by pathogens such as bacteria, viruses, accumulated food, chemical poisons or poisonous bites or stings. If not neutralized in the liver, such toxicity can accumulate and eventually pass to organs and tissues to produce symptoms such as fever, inflammation, infection, skin problems like acne and eczema, and sepsis. It can play a part in arthritis and is a factor in cancer and AIDS. The alterative action cools the blood either directly by killing the pathogens or indirectly by purifying and strengthening the liver and lymphatic system and by increasing the number and activity of the body's own immune cells. Demulcent alternatives like marshmallow root soothe irritations and counteract inflammations.

The Importance of Clean Blood

We instinctively know that good blood and blood circulation represent good health but rarely stop to think how accumulation of waste in the blood affects health. If waste and toxicity is not adequately removed from the blood and continues to circulate in the blood, it may be deposited in other tissues and become a focus of disease. Accumulation of waste is likely to impair tissue function and the blood flow may become sluggish so circulation is compromised and the heart must work harder to pump the blood around the body. In women during menses it can cause menstrual discomforts and because cells cannot receive their full requirement of oxygen and nutrients from congested blood, so their energy levels suffer. Blood purifying herbs help ensure clean vibrant blood which is crucial to health.

DIAPHORETIC ACTION

Examples: ginger, cayenne, sage, marjoram, hyssop, cinnamon, sassafras (warming diaphoretics). Yarrow, lemon balm, catnip, elderflower, peppermint, borage, chamomile, feverfew, chrysanthemum flowers (cooling diaphoretics).

Caution: while safe for occasional teas, culinary or short-term use, in pregnancy avoid prolonged or concentrated use of sage, peppermint, cayenne, marjoram, hyssop, cinnamon, sassafras. Avoid sassafras in conditions of strongly acute inflammation and for long-term use; avoid cayenne in presence of peptic ulcers and hyperthyroidism.

This action is also known as sudorific and these herbs promote sweating and the expulsion of toxicity through the skin. Diaphoretic herbs relieve surface fevers associated with common colds and flu, as well as coughs and mild asthma, skin eruptions, superficial oedema, body aches and stiffness, especially upper parts, arthritis, excess weight, swellings, and fluid retention. The herbs conduct the circulation of energy from the centre to the surface, and disperse stagnation. Their use is indicated for chills, colds and excess water, but the cooling ones are contraindicated for excess Air imbalances where the person, no matter what constitutional type, is weak and emaciated (dry and cold); and the warming ones are best avoided with very excessive heat or inflammatory conditions.

The Importance of Healthy Skin

The skin is not simply a covering for flesh and bones, but a major body organ as important as the liver, heart or lungs. Along with other functions, it provides immunity to infection and assists the elimination of waste. Like other parts of the body, the skin needs regular cleansing and nourishment. Several herbal remedies may be applied successfully through the skin, including teas, compresses, poultices and oils and creams in oleation therapy.

EXPECTORANT ACTION

Examples: thyme, licorice, comfrey leaves, hyssop, coltsfoot, mullein, basil, lungwort, white pine, elecampane, pleurisy root, kelp, eucalyptus, nettle, violet leaves.
Caution: licorice is avoided in water retention, oedema and cardiovascular conditions; elecampane and pleurisy root in pregnancy and kelp in hyperthyroidism, heart and kidney disease, TB and lung abscesses.

This action assists the body to remove excess phlegm, mucous or catarrh congesting the lungs, sinuses, and nasal passages and ears. Some expectorants help liquify and soften the phlegm and provide lubrication so that it is more easily expelled, some provide warmth to help dry and eliminate it and some stimulate elimination and disperse congestion.

Although manifesting in the lungs, a fundamental cause of acute excess mucous is most likely to lie in the stomach with poor digestion, and to fully resolve the situation herbal remedies would also include carminatives and circulatory stimulants. Avoiding mucous-forming foods such as dairy products, eggs, meat and refined flour products also helps.

Fire types or excess heat show signs such as inflammation with cloudy, yellow, fairly loose catarrh. Use cooling herbs such as comfrey, coltsfoot, pleurisy root, nettles, and violet leaves. Water types or excess Water show signs of sinus congestion, leading to headaches with clear, congesting phlegm. Use warming and/or drying herbs such as ginger, pepper or garlic combined with a carminative and a diuretic herb, to promote the elimination of excess damp. Air types or excess Air show a dry, or unproductive cough with fatigue, perhaps brought on by chill, stress or anxiety, fatigue. Use warming herbs combined with demulcent herbs to soften mucous and lubricate membranes and herbs to relax and nourish the nervous system (see Nervine Action p 44). In mixed types, choose herbs according to both symptoms and constitutional type. If there is inflammation, add anti-inflammatory and soothing herbs such as echinacea, slippery elm or marshmallow root.

Whenever there are symptoms of blood in the sputum, extreme dryness in nose and throat, continued or repeated fever or inflammation, or weakness, fatigue, and a thin watery mucous discharge, these indicate a more complex and deeper problem and professional advice should be sought.

The Importance of Healthy Lungs

Breathing is an involuntary bodily activity that we tend to take for granted, and the lungs may take a lot of pounding before they show noticeable signs of stress. The energy derived from air is vital for the health of each body cell and its processes.

A deficiency of oxygen and incomplete elimination of carbonic wastes via the lungs can leave the Vital Force weakened and congested. It is not a good idea to put up with congested sinuses and lungs, considering them to be only minor conditions, as the congestion will continually drain the body's energy bit by bit. The use of lung-clearing herbs can clear blockages and maintain the health of lung tissue and a few minutes of full, deep breathing, practised daily with a calm, relaxed mind will revitalize and bring balance.

DIURETIC ACTION

Examples: chickweed, juniper berries, cleavers, horsetail, parsley, couch grass, fennel, shepherd's purse, plantain, yarrow, marsh-mallow, dandelion, fenugreek, raspberry.
Caution: while safe for occasional teas, culinary or short-term use, in pregnancy avoid prolonged or concentrated use of parsley, juniper and fenugreek. Avoid shepherd's purse in hyper-thyroidism.

This action benefits the urinary system, improving the excretion of urine but at the same time nourishing the urinary organs and promoting balanced water and mineral metabolism at cellular level. Common ailments of the urinary system include kidney stones, cystitis, urinary tract infections, painful burning sensations, swelling of the prostate, excess uric acid, incontinence and retention of urine. Even lower back ache may be related to poor kidney function.

The Importance of Kidney Function

The kidneys perform the important jobs of cleansing the blood, adjusting the fluid and electrolyte balance in the body, and helping to regulate blood pressure. Connected to the Water element, they symbolize the basic fluid milieu from which life and growth arise and by which they are sustained. Poor function of the kidneys can be a factor in such conditions as oedema, lymphatic congestion, excess weight, menstrual congestion, and in respiratory, skin and liver complaints. Herbs will simultaneously nourish and strengthen the function of the organs, and raise the health of the body generally. Juniper is not recommended in the presence of inflammation of the kidneys.

BLOOD REGULATING AND EMMENAGOGUE ACTION

Examples: angelica, dong quai, shepherd's purse, myrrh, turmeric, garlic, thyme, marjoram, squaw vine, raspberry, yarrow, motherwort, cayenne, hawthorn berries, comfrey leaves.

Caution: While safe for occasional use in pregnancy, avoid concentrated or prolonged use of thyme, marjoram, garlic, cayenne; avoid angelica and dong quai altogether. Avoid dong quai in presence of diarrhoea or abdominal fullness.

This action affects the circulation and movement of blood, the liquid tissue of the body, promoting its efficient, smooth and correctly channelled flow. When there is either congestion or injury to the body, this will in some way affect the blood flow, causing either stagnation or haemorrhaging. Therapeutic blood regulating action helps with blood or circulation problems – such as menstrual irregularity or discomfort, anaemia, weakness, cold, stroke or hypertension – as well as trauma to tissues from wounds, sprains or operations. It promotes healing, prevents sepsis and clears the bruising.

Warming blood regulators include thyme, angelica, garlic, turmeric, myrrh and dong quai; cooling ones include comfrey, motherwort, yarrow, shepherd's purse and raspberry. Tonifying blood regulators include nettles, dong quai, yarrow and myrrh; raspberry is particularly tonifying to the uterus. Relaxing ones include dong quai, angelica, thyme, marjoram and shepherd's purse. Herbs to arrest bleeding include cayenne, comfrey, shepherd's purse and turmeric.

Blood Regulators for Women

Blood regulatory herbs are used for both sexes but they are especially important for women, as female physiology is intimately connected to the quality of blood and the circulation of bodily fluids and hormones. Premenstrual tension (PMT) for example, is a sign of disharmony and rather than accepting this as inevitable, it is better to respond to the sign positively in order to resolve the imbalance.

At menstruation, the body – at all levels, physical, emotional and mental – shows whether it is in healthy state of balance or not. Feelings of depression, irritability or vulnerability around this time can be caused by physical congestion of fluids. Also, the body can use the monthly flow as an extra pathway of elimination. The uterus, ovaries or vagina may become the site of infections, polyps, cysts or discharges as the body tries to cope with the toxicity. Depression or severe discomforts during the menstrual cycle may recur at the menopause so correcting imbalances and sorting out problems early may save discomfort later. To be reasonably in balance means less physical discomfort, and many women feel more creative or insightful around this time.

DEMULCENT ACTION

Examples: marshmallow root, kelp, slippery elm, licorice, kudzu, oats, fenugreek, flax, chickweed, clover, mullein, comfrey, coltsfoot, fennel.
Caution: avoid fenugreek and fennel in pregnancy, except for occasional, short-term use. Avoid kelp in hyperthyroidism, heart and kidney disease, TB and lung abcesses. Avoid licorice in water retention, oedema, cardiovascular disease.

This action has a very special quality to it: as these herbs combine with water they become moist, soft and dense and when they meet body tissue they impart these qualities to it and soothe irritated, inflamed, swollen, 'angry' tissue – whether externally as a skin problem, or internally as perhaps an irritable bowel. They calm inordinate heat of urinary infections, burns or sore throats, and sweet, moistening herbs like licorice and red clover will nourish the Water essence needed in cases of extreme dryness, wasting, emaciation, weakness or fatigue.

ASTRINGENT ACTION

Examples: mullein, raspberry, eyebright, oak bark, squaw vine, pine, comfrey, shepherd's purse, sage, golden seal.

This action has a condensing, tightening and drying effect on tissues, and is commonly used to treat symptoms of acute fluid elimination such as runny or bleeding noses, diarrhoea, internal and external bleeding, discharge of pus, and vaginal discharge. It is also used to tone flaccid muscles, mucous membranes or cell walls. Symptomatic treatment should always be combined with herbs to redress the underlying causes of the condition.

NERVINE ACTION

Examples: skullcap, lemon balm, catnip, wood betony, passion flower, valerian, chamomile, ginger, thyme, vervain, wild yam. *Caution*: while safe for occasional use, avoid prolonged or concentrated use of thyme and vervain in pregnancy.

This action affects the nervous system and through it the entire body. Nervine herbs are antispasmodic and release muscular tension, both conscious and unconscious, reduce and relieve pain by their analgesic and sedative action, and calm nerves and induce relaxation and sleep. Some nervines can nourish nerve tissues, strengthening the system generally and counteracting stress. Some have a lightening quality that lifts lowered spirits while calming anxiety, and some an earthy quality which grounds nervous excitability and spaciness.

The Importance of Healthy Nerves

It has been estimated that about 75 per cent of all disease is due in part to stress which affects primarily the nervous and endocrine systems. The nervous system relates directly to the Air element. Feelings of isolation, anxiety, ungroundedness, or physical symptoms of spasm, pain and tension show the involvement of the nerves and endocrine glands. (For further information see *The Stress of Life* by Hans Seyle). Residual tension can be locked in the body although we may be unaware of it and regularly finding a space of utter calmness, a point of stillness with a minimum of mental and physical activity, allows the body to recuperate, to re-align itself, reintegrate, and balance the flow of the deepest, rhythmic pulsations of the Life Force.

TONIFYING ACTION

Examples: ginseng, dong quai, raspberry, oats, red clover, golden seal, garlic, ginger, licorice, asparagus root, fenugreek, walnuts, celery seeds, juniper berries, slippery elm, comfrey leaves, irish moss, sesame seeds, marshmallow root, Solomon's seal, molasses, almonds, honey, jujube dates, saw palmetto, thyme, yellow gentian. *Caution*: while safe for occasional short-term use, in pregnancy avoid concentrated or prolonged use of juniper, garlic and fenugreek. Avoid altogether dong quai, ginseng and golden seal in pregnancy. Avoid licorice in water retention, oedema and cardiovascular disease. Avoid asparagus in diarrhoea.

This action includes more than may at first be apparent. In addition to strengthening individual organs and tissues, tonifying restores the body generally to strength and vitality and, used regularly, maintains a vibrant level. By nourishing tissues and energy it helps combat disease, increases immunity and enhances the quality of life. Though historically the art of tonification therapy is perhaps not as fully developed in western herbal medicine, our own western herbs are now being successfully used for the purpose.

Tonifying herbs are especially indicated where there is emaciation, debility, or weakness but the more assertive ones such as ginseng or juniper are avoided during an acute crisis such as a fever, infection, inflammation, cold or flu because the strength of the herb will tend to add strength to the illness.

WOUND HEALING ACTION

Examples: marigold, slippery elm, lemon balm, comfrey leaves, plantain, yarrow, walnut leaves, witch hazel, aloe, lavender.

This action promotes the regrowth of new cells and healing of traumatized tissue. The herbs have soothing, antiseptic, astringent and blood regulating properties – bringing blood to the site when needed but also preventing haemorrhaging and blood stasis. Used internally as well as externally, they heal bruises and abrasions and deeper traumatized tissues such as sprains, torn ligaments, dry or emaciated tissue, weakened vertebrae and broken bones.

THE SUBTLE THERAPEUTIC EFFECTS OF HERBS

When you have been using herbs for a while either as a regular part of keeping yourself well or as medicine during an illness, when you have handled them in preparing teas or perhaps in growing them as beautiful plants in the garden, you eventually

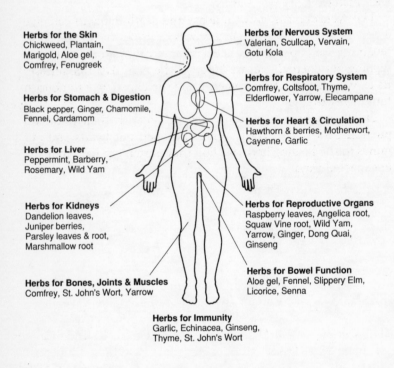

Herbs for the Skin
Chickweed, Plantain, Marigold, Aloe gel, Comfrey, Fenugreek

Herbs for Stomach & Digestion
Black pepper, Ginger, Chamomile, Fennel, Cardamom

Herbs for Liver
Peppermint, Barberry, Rosemary, Wild Yam

Herbs for Kidneys
Dandelion leaves, Juniper berries, Parsley leaves & root, Marshmallow root

Herbs for Bones, Joints & Muscles
Comfrey, St. John's Wort, Yarrow

Herbs for Nervous System
Valerian, Scullcap, Vervain, Gotu Kola

Herbs for Respiratory System
Comfrey, Coltsfoot, Thyme, Elderflower, Yarrow, Elecampane

Herbs for Heart & Circulation
Hawthorn & berries, Motherwort, Cayenne, Garlic

Herbs for Reproductive Organs
Raspberry leaves, Angelica root, Squaw Vine root, Wild Yam, Yarrow, Ginger, Dong Quai, Ginseng

Herbs for Bowel Function
Aloe gel, Fennel, Slippery Elm, Licorice, Senna

Herbs for Immunity
Garlic, Echinacea, Ginseng, Thyme, St. John's Wort

Figure 2   Herbs for Organs and Systems

become aware that they are having an unexpected effect on your life.

In using herbs medicinally, you are connecting with the fundamental energies of nature, of the earth, of the seasons and the weather. You are interacting with your environment, rather than just passing through life living in protective bubbles of convenience, distracting entertainments and stimulations. Using herbs engages you in communication with your self, leads to more self-awareness and challenges you to learn. It may happen that you notice you have a particular affinity for one or more herbs. You may be drawn to them because of their colour, taste, form, by some association, or through seeing a particularly beautiful or interesting plant in a garden or in the wild. One or two herbs may seem to work better than others for a particular ailment to which you are especially prone. It's lovely to develop such a relationship with plants.

The cycle of birth, growth, decay and death in plants can give a new perspective to the same processes in our own lives. How much are we clinging to what has turned into a burden for us, sapping our energy? Can we let go of the past, as a tree releases its leaves when the time comes, using the experience to nourish future growth?

Plants are quietly, modestly getting on with their lives and providing for our survival. When we open our hearts and our minds to the healing herbs we find they enrich our lives in many unexpected ways.

5

Hands-on Herbs

GATHERING YOUR HERBS

W ANDERING THE COUNTRY lanes or forests, or walking through
a garden gathering herbs, is a delight and adventure as
well as a restoring of the soul – a therapy in itself. Practically,
however, there are several factors to consider before starting out
and a little preparation will save both your time and the viability
of the plants you are seeking.

Cautions and Precautions

Gathering herbs in the wild can present a problem where
population density is high and agriculture, industry or traffic is
intensive for the herbs are likely to have become contaminated
with chemical pollutants. A good rule of thumb is to gather from
a site at least a hundred yards or around ninety metres from the
nearest main road or field, and several miles from an industrial
site. One solution may be to gather from the waysides around an
organic garden, having obtained permission of course.

Remember to dress according to the weather or terrain: wear
protective clothing and gloves if necessary; carry a basket or large
bag and some secateurs. A strong root stick or garden fork for
digging roots and a small axe if cutting bark will be needed.

Handling some herbs such as yarrow or St John's wort in
quantity may provoke an allergic skin or respiratory reaction in
a few individuals. This is entirely unpredictable as it depends on
an idiosyncratic response or the amount handled, but if you are

prone to this, take precautions by wearing gloves or a nose mask while gathering herbs.

Responsible Gathering

The demand for herbs is growing with the popularity of herbal medicine, and all herbs should be gathered wild from uncontaminated sites, but in fact this poses many problems – the most important being that it can threaten the very existence of some species. *The European Journal of Herbal Medicine* reports that since 1982 over a hundred tonnes of dried herbs have been imported into Britain from the US each year; 250 tonnes in 1992 alone. As only a few of these herbs are grown commercially on any scale, the rest must have been harvested wild. In North America, population pressure, the gathering of ginseng, golden seal, and *Trillium* since the eighteenth and nineteenth centuries and now echinacea in the twentieth has already greatly reduced the range of these herbs. Similar situations already exist, or soon will, in other countries. When buying over-the-counter products, it is a good idea to enquire how the raw materials are obtained to encourage the organic cultivation of plants. For personal use, avoid collecting from any but the most common plants and if you are in any doubt consult your local nature conservancy association. Even excluding the rarer species, there is still a very large number of plants that can be safely harvested from the wild and are well worth the effort, many of them our most common weeds. 'Wild crafting', a term which has sprung up in America, captures the spirit of this aspect of herbal medicine. It indicates that collecting and preparing herbs is a skill involving considerable knowledge, thoughtfulness and craft. In a way it connects us full circle with the itinerant rhizomatists of ancient Greece – literally the root vendors – who gathered and prepared herbs for the people.

Guidelines for Gathering Plants

Mindfulness

The best way to go about gathering is to adopt the practice of the Native Americans. When gathering, they take only from a place where the plant is growing in profusion and, before cutting, they pause and offer words of appreciation and thanks to the plant and to the spirit for the healing gift within it. They never take more than one third of the plants within a group, nor more than one third of each particular plant, unless it is a single rooted plant like dandelion. This is a beautiful meditation practice, involving humility and consideration for the good of the plant and its habitat, and acknowledging the cosmic healing force in nature. It subtly enhances the healing power of the herbs so gathered.

Practicalities

Identification
Whether in the wild or the garden be sure you can accurately identify the exact species of the plants you want. Take a good identification guide along, and if there is any doubt, do not gather. Observe carefully and only collect from plants that are healthy, in good condition, and free of chemical pollution.

Timing
Give thought to the weather, the time of day and the season of the year. However climates, weather conditions and seasons vary greatly all over the world and even from year to year so it is not practical to try to learn specific times. Gathering herbs involves being attuned with the local environment and following a few general principles.

● Gather your herbs in when the plants are dry – that is, not after a rain or in heavy dew.

● Gather plant parts before the sun is at its height, especially when gathering aromatic parts, as the sun's warmth will at first draw out but later reduce the aromatic molecules as it gets hotter.

● Gather the desired plant part in which the medicinal properties are most concentrated (indicated in the Materia medica) when it is at its peak. To follow this it is helpful to imagine the sap or life blood of the plant as it flows through the tissues, from the root through to seed formation; it rises in spring from winter hibernation and gradually quickens each part of the plant. So for example, early spring is the best time to collect the medicinal roots or rhizomes, such as dandelion, burdock, elecampane, yellow dock and angelica. If you miss these roots in the spring you do get a second chance in the autumn when the aerial parts die and the sap returns to the roots for winter. Some plants mature quickly and their tender young leaves are also available in spring, making it the ideal time for the collection of herbs such as nettles, dandelion leaves, coltsfoot and comfrey leaves.

• If gathering the leaves and flowering stem, or the flower itself, collect them when they are fresh. The leaves of some plants, such as lavender, lemon balm, hyssop, rosemary and sage, are collected just before the plant flowers. Sometimes it is only the flowering heads that are wanted and as these continue to flower they can be gathered periodically. Such herbs include marigold, rose and borage. Pick the flowers just as they are opening fully.

• If the properties you require are concentrated in the seeds or fruit, collect in late summer or autumn when they are ripe; for example fennel seeds, hawthorn berries and rose hips.

• Collecting medicinal barks from shrubs and trees such as peach, slippery elm and cramp bark (guelder rose) is done when the sap has just come into that part, either in spring when it is rising or in autumn when it is flowing back towards the root.

These collection times are when the life energy of the plant is at its most expressive or developed and the therapeutic properties most concentrated. But what if you have missed this ideal time or need the plant immediately and the perfect conditions are not there, does this mean it is not worth collecting and using the herb? Not at all. It is fine to gather it then and there, whether it is at its height or not. Freshness counts for a lot and you need not avoid collecting a herb just because the conditions were not ideal.

Some traditional healers gather according to intuition. For example if, among all the plants that are good for wounds – comfrey, mullein, plantain, St John's Wort or yarrow – you look about you and instinctively feel that one of these is right for that particular person with that particular wound, you would be justified in collecting it for use.

Others value where the plant grows: if it survives in harsher conditions, on the north side of a mountain for example, or in poor soil, its energy may be that much stronger, even though it may not be as large or lush as one growing in a warm valley.

Procedure

Having chosen the specimen, and the time and place for collecting, use the following guidelines for harvesting.

● Only gather from places where there is an abundance of the plant. Do not take more than you need and never more than one small amount of the population. Never gather from a plant that is a threatened or protected species.

● When gathering the aerial parts, only cut them from the top one-third of the stem and never take more than one-third of the stems or flowers. For roots, it is of course necessary to dig the whole root. For seeds, it is best to cut the stem just below the seed head and take it home intact. Flowering heads may be cut just beneath the florets.

● Always collect bark from a branch, not the main trunk, and never remove the bark in a full circle around it. Instead, cut a rectangular area of the outer bark about one-third of the way around and remove this. Alternatively cut a branch that must be pruned anyway, then scrape off or cut away just the inner, living cambium layer; do not go deeply into the tree. An alternative is to collect the twigs and small branches of the tree in spring when the sap has risen, as if pruning the tree. Take the inner bark and cut it up before drying.

● When taking the inner bark of roots, having gathered them whole, scrape away the thin outer layer and collect the inner bark.

PROCESSING YOUR HERBS

Begin the storing process immediately, if the herbs are not to be consumed there and then. Two things are needed to preserve herbs at their best: dehydration to remove all traces of moisture, and careful storage to protect from light, damp and heat.

Drying (Dehydration)

Gently shake, brush or wash away any trace of dirt, dust or insects, and dry any remaining damp. Then proceed with the correct method according to which particular parts you are drying.

Roots and bark

Chop these into small pieces before drying to speed dehydration and make them easier to handle later. Lay pieces out on a tray or cloth away from direct light in a warm place such as the airing cupboard, the top of a boiler, or near a wood stove. To dry more quickly, place the herbs in a warm oven on the very lowest setting, warming the oven, then turning off the heat and reheating briefly and periodically to maintain the lowest temperature.

Leaves and flowering stems

Tie these in small bundles at the base and hang them upside down in a warm, dry, airy place, out of light, where the air can circulate freely around them. Protect them from dust by placing under a muslin cloth, or in a paper bag with holes punched in. When dry, spread out a large clean cloth or piece of paper to catch the leaves or flowers as you rub or cut them off. Light stems may be kept and chopped into small pieces.

Flowering heads

Place on a tray or on a cloth stretched across a frame and keep in a warm dark place. Check them frequently and turn them to speed up the drying process. When dry, the flowers may be rubbed gently to break them into smaller pieces, especially if they are to be put into mixtures.

Fruit

Either keep on the stem, hang up as for leaves and remove when dry, or remove individual fruits carefully and dry as for root pieces. Fruit peel may be stripped and chopped before drying as for roots.

Seeds

Dry the seed head whole, hanging it by the stem. When dry, lay out a large, clean sheet of paper or cloth and shake the seed heads and/or rub them over it. Alternatively, remove the seeds when first collected over the sheet, then spread them on a tray to dry in a warm place away from light.

Completing the drying

The test for the completion of the drying process is to feel the material; it should feel crisp and dry, and crumble or break easily with a snap. The time this takes will depend entirely on the conditions and method used but regular, periodic checking will monitor progress.

Storing Your Herbs

While herbs will keep for several years in the right conditions, it is best to gather them freshly and dry them each year, especially in the case of aromatic ones. Once dried, herbs may be placed in any clean, dry container made of glass, wood, papier mâché, or a household tin with a tight fitting lid. Identify and date the herbs with a label on the container. It's also nice to record where they were collected as a reminder. Store the containers away from heat and direct sunlight. Using decorative labels with handsome lettering means the containers can be attractively displayed in a dark side of the room.

USING YOUR HERBS: PREPARATIONS AND METHODS OF APPLICATION

There are many different ways of taking herbs, from simply eating them raw as a nourishing supplement to brewing a delicious aromatic tea or applying them as an oil or ointment. The kitchen becomes a veritable pharmacy in itself! The therapeutic effect you desire determines the choice of preparation and whether it is applied internally or externally.

Infusions and Decoctions

An infusion, or herbal tea, is made with the lighter, more delicate or aerial parts of a plant – the leaves, flowers, and non-woody stems – and may be taken internally or applied externally. Medicinal strength tea is made with one cup of water for each teaspoon of dried herbs or two teaspoons of fresh herbs and brewed at least fifteen minutes. Make as for any pot of tea by boiling the water, warming the pot or pan, steeping the well-covered herbs and straining. Use only ceramic, stainless steel or glass containers, never metals like aluminium.

If taking many cups of tea in a day, you may make a large amount and store it in the fridge or a cool place. Gently rewarm on *very* low heat if it is to be taken warm. Some teas are taken cool. Another way to make herb tea is to steep the herbs cold in water overnight or through a day, especially in a sunny spot.

When the medicinal properties of a plant are concentrated in its tougher parts – the inner bark, roots, rhizomes, woody stems or seeds – they are extracted by a decoction. The proportions are the same as for an infusion but instead of brewing, a decoction slowly simmers in a closed pan for about fifteen to twenty minutes. Again, always use glass, enamel or stainless steel, never aluminium, brass, copper, or non-stick-coated pans. If the tougher parts can be ground to a powder first, then they can be brewed as an infusion.

Externally, infusions and decoctions, referred to here as tea, are used in a number of ways.

Inhalations

Prepare a tea with the appropriate aromatic herbs. Pour the tea into a basin, place a large towel over the head, bend over the basin, enclosing your face in the steam with the towel. Breathe calmly, inhaling the aromatic steam. At intervals, pause for ordinary breathing. Repeat four or five times or until relieved.

Washes

Herbal teas can be used to bathe a local area of skin affected by, for example, skin eruptions, itching or inflammation. They may be used to bathe the body during a fever, and for hair rinses.

Foot- and hand-baths

This method was used extensively by the French herbalist Maurice Messegué to great effect. He prescribed warm foot-or hand-baths for 8 minutes, morning and evening. The healing principles in the herbs are absorbed through the skin and circulated throughout the body. This can be a very effective treatment and an alternative for those who dislike the taste of a particular herb. Prepare enough tea to cover the foot or hand to the ankle or wrist, as hot as is comfortable.

Fomentations

Cloths are soaked in the prepared herbal tea, wrung out and applied to the affected body part, either warm or cool as required. Fomentations are applied to local areas of inflammation, itching, eruptions or pain: arthritis, rheumatism, bursitis, boils, psoriasis, eczema, sprained muscles and ligaments, joint aches and lower back pain. If heat is needed, as happens with dull aches and soreness, replace the cloth as it cools with one freshly soaked in hot tea; include warming herbs in the blend – ginger or pepper. For inflammatory states, cool fomentations can be applied and left overnight; cover with a piece of clingfilm and bind comfortably in place.

Tinctures

These are like cold infusions of herbs but instead of using water as solvent, spirits such as brandy or vodka (60% proof) are used. The spirits act as preservatives so herbs can be on hand for use at any time. In some herbs, a therapeutic constituent may not be soluble in water, so a tea form of the herb is less effective; a spirit contains both alcohol and water so all the properties are obtained and will pass more quickly into the circulation when in tincture form. Disadvantages are taste, for those who do not like alcohol, and the effect on the liver for those with a history of liver weakness or alcoholism. Tinctures may also be made with apple-cider vinegar.

To prepare a tincture, use a clean, wide-mouth large jar with a tight-fitting lid. Chop the chosen herbs beforehand or use powders. Combine 1 pt (570 ml) of vodka with 4 oz (113g) of dried herb, 8 oz (227g) of fresh herb, in the jar. Cap the jar tightly and place in a spot you will be passing frequently, away from direct sunlight. Shake the tincture at least three times a day. A good idea is to stick on a big label saying SHAKE ME, to remind any passers-by. Macerate (soak) the tincture in this way for two weeks, then strain away the herbs and bottle the tincture in a brown-glass container, such as a wine bottle or one obtained from the chemist. Seal with a wax-coated cork or tight cap. Many people like to start tinctures when there is a new moon and bottle them on the full moon, feeling that the drawing power of the moon as it waxes increases the potency of the medicine.

An example of a useful tincture is catnip and fennel. Made with equal parts of catnip leaves and fennel seeds, it is excellent for an upset stomach, especially one due to nervousness and anxiety, or for calming and soothing at any time. It is good for children's tummy upsets, diluted with water.

Liniments

These are made exactly like tinctures. They are for external use as muscle rubs, or for applying to cuts and wounds. Apple-cider vinegar is a good medium, as is surgical spirit. Good herbs to use are warming, penetrating and antiseptic ones such as ginger, eucalyptus, cayenne or black pepper, and myrrh; or cooling, healing, astringent ones such as golden seal, marigold, St John's wort and comfrey leaf which also make good aftershave washes.

Jethro Kloss' liniment comes in handy for many conditions such as muscle strain, sprain, wounds and arthritic joints. Make it with 2 parts myrrh, 1 part cayenne and 1 part golden seal.

Syrups

Syrups are made for coughs, sore throats and respiratory conditions. First brew a strong herb tea then mix with an equal amount of honey, or glycerine. Another method is to concentrate the herbal tea by simmering it down slowly to half its original amount and then adding raw, brown sugar or honey to thicken. Herbs such as thyme, violet leaves, sage, garlic and licorice all make good syrups. Store in the refrigerator for up to a week.

Poultices

This treatment, like liniments and fomentations, is a local external application and used for the same types of conditions. Poultices are valuable for first aid to wounds and burns, even major ones. They are excellent for traumatized vertebrae, broken bones and torn muscles and ligaments.

Cut a clean cotton cloth twice the size of the area you want to cover. Blend the selected herbs either dried, fresh (chopped small) or powdered. Include a herb like slippery elm or a small amount of flour, cornflour (starch) or cornmeal to act as a binding agent and give bulk. Place the herbs on the cloth and the cloth on a plate or shallow bowl. Pour on just enough boiled water to moisten and create a thick mass. Wrap the sides around the herbs, and place the poultice, warm or cool as needed, on the area to be covered. Cover with clingfilm to retain moisture and with a thick towel or blanket to retain heat. Replace as needed. Poultices may be left on overnight.

When away from home an instant poultice may be made by chewing the leaves of helpful wound herbs found in the location and applying the pulp formed straight onto the skin. Such herbs would include chickweed, plantain, comfrey, yarrow and woundwort.

Oils and Ointments

Herbal oils can be used for salad dressings, for massage and for muscle rubs, ear aches, as well as for nourishing enemas. Healing ointments are easily made from herbal oils by simply adding beeswax, or cocoa butter. Aromatherapy massage oils may be made from your own garden herbs such as lavender, rosemary, thyme, St. John's wort and mint. Ginger and garlic make useful oils.

To make a herbal oil, fill a wide-mouth jar with 1 pt (570 ml) of any good light vegetable oil, such as grapeseed, soy or sunflower, preferably cold-pressed. Add 2 1/2 oz. (70 g) of dried herb (50oz/140g of fresh), cover tightly and macerate in a warm place for three days. Strain away the herb and bottle the oil in sterile bottles. To make a stronger oil, replace with more herb and repeat as desired. When the oil is needed right away, warm herbs in oil gently on a low flame for an hour; strain. Store oils in a cool place.

To make a healing ointment for the first aid kit, prepare a herbal oil as above using comfrey leaves, chickweed, calendula, plaintain or yarrow. Warm the strained oil; grate in one or more ounces of beeswax or cocoa butter, stirring until melted. Test for consistency by coating a spoon; it should solidify within moments. Add more beeswax if necessary. Pour into sterilized jars and cap.

The Herbal Bolus

The bolus is a type of poultice applied internally to the vaginal area. It is useful for drawing toxins from the reproductive area and healing the local tissues. These are best used under the guidance of a qualified herbalist, though a simple one can be made with slippery elm powder. Warm some coconut oil to melt and mix in the herb to form a thick paste. Cool, then shape into an index-finger-sized cylinder; when solid again, cut into 1 in (2.5 cm) pieces and place one to three of these into the vagina. Cover the entrance with a cut-off tampon and use a sanitary towel to protect clothing. Leave on overnight and remove the next day. Douche with warm, boiled water or herbal tea. Repeat as needed.

The Herbal Enema

Unfortunately enemas have a bad reputation due to the over-zealous fanaticism of our Victorian predecessors. However they have an important role to play in healing and the therapy is not unpleasant when performed willingly and with understanding. Used periodically as part of internal body cleansing, enema therapy maintains the health of the bowel, prevents the build-up of toxicity there, ar.d regulates the Air humour. During an acute crisis, such as a fever, it can quickly remove toxins from the body and relieve symptoms. Enemas are beneficial in cases of constipation, candida, parasites, arthritis and rheumatism, fevers, leucorrhoea, nervousness and irritability. Enemas are important in the Gerson cancer-therapy programme. Both herbal oils and teas are used, chosen according to the symptoms and the humoural balance of the person. In cases of inability to digest or even to eat, enemas can be life saving, as nourishment can be provided to the body indirectly by nourishing the tissues via enemas of herbs and strained gruels – an integral part of Ayurvedic therapeutics.

Purchase an enema kit with a tube which can be easily opened and closed. Prepare 2 pt (1140 ml) of the appropriate herb tea or oil and keep it warm. Fill the container first with tepid salt water. Lie down on a large towel on the floor of a warm bathroom with knees bent toward the chest and suspend the bottle 3 ft (0.9m) above you.

Grease the tip of the tube with some oil and insert it into the rectum, release the opening and allow the tepid water to enter the colon. When it begins to feel full, close the opening and allow the liquid to be absorbed. Repeat until 1 pt (570 ml) or more of water has been held, proceeding slowly at the pace that is comfortable for you. To encourage absorption, lie first on your left side and then on the right; gently massage the abdomen from left to right. Void the solution after about ten to twenty minutes.

Now repeat the procedure using the herbal oil or tea. You may not be able to retain the full amount the first time, but as the therapy is repeated – up to twice in a week is sufficient – you will be able to retain more as the colon is cleansed. For health maintenance, use enema therapy once a month, or during one week every spring and autumn. If used during an acute crisis, such as a fever, return to bedrest immediately after completion.

Pills and Capsules

This is a convenient, tasteless, way to take herbs that involves the least processing, so is closer to raw form. Many herbs can be powdered finely enough in the coffee-grinding attachment of a home blender.

To make pills, mix 1–2 tablespoons of honey for 1 oz (28g) of herb; the amount of honey varies with the texture of the herbs. Add a small amount of boiled water gradually until the powder thickens to a dough-like consistency; adding a little slippery elm powder or flour will help this. Roll the dough into a ball and pinch off small amounts; roll between your fingers to the shape and size of a pea. Flatten these between your fingers and place on a baking tray. Warm in a very slow oven until the moisture is removed. Store the pills in an airtight jar and keep in the refrigerator. The honey will act as a preservative.

To fill capsules, obtain some gelatine capsules from a health-food shop or chemist. Place the powdered herbs in a bowl. Take each capsule and separate, then tap each end in the powder to fill before replacing the ends together. This is very time-consuming but in some places a home capsuling gadget is commercially available.

The Herbal Pillow

Elizabeth Hayes, a Wiltshire herbalist, has extended the use of the traditional herbal pillow from just a sleeping aid to therapy for almost any ailment. This is a good example of how herbs heal by their vibrational energy, for not all the herbs used in the pillows are aromatic. Her pillows have successfully treated conditions ranging from pre-menstrual tension to asthma. They are especially good for children.

Choose the dried herbs for your condition. Cut a small muslin cloth about nine inches square. Place the herbs inside and sew it up. Cover with another cloth of attractive print, if desired. Place the pillow inside your pillow case and the healing energies will do their work while you sleep. Renew the pillow at least annually.

The Herbal Bath and Sweating Therapy

Sweat baths for sweating therapy have been used as an important method of curing disease and maintaining health in cultures from Native American to Indian. Sweat baths also have a spiritual purpose in such traditions because a clean, healthy body is considered analogous or preparatory to a purified mind and consciousness receptive to enlightenment.

As more and more spas, gyms and health clubs are beginning to offer saunas and steam baths, it is possible for many people to make use of sweating therapy for maintaining health. (Be sure to take your diaphoretic herbal tea with you in a thermos flask to drink.) However, for those who do not have such a facility, the therapy may be adapted and performed in the home as a herbal bath and sweat to cleanse the body of impurities.

Sweating is good for skin problems, and conditions of excess weight or toxicity, for the first signs of cold or flu, and for routine cleansing. Sweating promotes elimination through the skin of the toxins, or the chill which may have provoked the cold or fever. When ill, it helps if a friend or family member can assist you. A sweat will benefit any of the three humoural types in those of basically sound health but is especially indicated for Water type persons who are overweight or prone to excess mucous conditions or arthritis.

PLEASE NOTE: Sweating therapy is contraindicated for any one who has high blood pressure, hepatitis or jaundice; is thin, weak, anaemic, or emaciated; is suffering from shock, grief or an extreme emotional state; and for pregnant women.

Procedure for home sweating therapy

Brew a large and strong pot of diaphoretic and warming herbs, chosen according to your constitutional type. Three herbs combined give a better effect. Draw as hot a bath as comfortable for you and throw in two handfuls of Epsom salts for extra cleansing: they help draw toxins out through the skin. Fill one or two hot-water bottles, or turn on an electric blanket and place in your bed; add extra blankets or quilts.

Pour the herb tea into the bath water, reserving a cup or two to drink while in the bath. A few drops of essential oils may be added to the bath water to enhance the process. Close off the bath with a shower curtain if possible. Keep the head, and genitals of males, cool with a cold damp cloth. Drink your tea, then relax and absorb the herbs. You may begin to perspire in the bath, which is a good sign.

After soaking for 15–20 minutes, and while still hot, get out of the bath, pat yourself only lightly dry and go straight to bed with the hot-water bottles and warm bedclothes. Rest or sleep (overnight is fine), while keeping very warm and the body should perspire or sweat. When you wake, rinse or sponge off with tepid water mixed with half the amount of cider vinegar. You will feel amazingly refreshed and clean. For a stubborn cold or flu, repeat the sweat the next day.

DOSAGES

The effects of herbs depends to an extent on how often they are taken. For acute ailments, in general it is best to take the herbs quite frequently, every hour or even half hour, until some relief appears in the symptoms. Then continue the dose at gradually longer intervals up to two or three times a day until the condition clears.

Herb teas and decoctions

Adults should take 1 cup every hour or so to relieve symptoms for short-term, acute conditions then 1 cup three times a day for follow-up or longer-term treatment.

Capsules or pills

Adults take 2 capsules or 4 pills every hour as needed in acute conditions, or three times a day with meals for follow-up and longer-term treatment.

Tinctures

Adults take 1 tsp or 5ml every hour as needed, or three times a day for follow-up or longer-term treatment.

Poultices or external applications

Judge according to the situation, and use the same general guideline – apply frequently until relieved, then less often.

Long-term imbalances

For imbalances that have been present for some time, though are not manifesting acutely at the moment, dosage would be 1 cup, 1 tsp or 2 capsules three times a day for three weeks. Rest one week, then re-assess, and repeat if needed.

Children

For children, the adult dose is reduced proportionately according to age; this is based on weight, so make adjustments if the child is not average weight for age. Dilute with water or juice.

- Nursing infants – mother to take the herbs. Their effects will pass through the milk to the baby.
- 6mth – 1 year: 1/8 or less (depending on weight) of adult dose
- 1–2 years: 1/4 of adult dose
- 3–7 years: 1/2 of adult dose
- 7–12 years: 3/4 of adult dose

Elderly

For elderly patients, adjust the dose according to how frail they are. If they are hardy and sturdy, even if old, the adult dose can apply. If frail and weak, use the doses for small children under seven.

USING YOUR HERBS

Once the herbs have been gathered, processed and stored they are ready to put to use. The best results come when herbs are matched to the constitutional temperament of the person and the pattern of the ailment, and chosen to balance any aggravated or weak state and maintain the natural balance.

When choosing which herbs to use decide which therapeutic action or combination of actions will best support the body's own healing activity. Refer to Chapter 3 and consult the Humour Assessment table on page 32, and the Using Your Herbs table on page 68. Information on individual herbs is found in the Materia Medica of this or other more detailed books. When deciding which herbs to use you will be also guided to some extent by what is available to you at the time – it may be the middle of the night when you need them! Remember that several herbs can be used for the same condition, so that if you don't have the particular one that is recommended, don't worry: choose ones with similar therapeutic properties that you do have.

Next, consider which method to use to apply the herbs: for

example whether internally as a tea or decoction or externally as a poultice or compress, and whether to take them hot, warm or cool. Base your choice on the location and strength of the ailment and the energy pattern of the person; and it may be that a combination of treatments is needed. For example, for a cold you could drink herb teas, soak in a herb bath or footbath, breathe a herbal steam, *and* take garlic pills.

Energetic Treatment with Herbs

In general, excess Fire needs herbs with cooling energy to reduce excess heat and only mildly warming energy herbs to enhance elimination. Fire can also be dispersed through the skin with diaphoretic herbs and sweating therapy. Excess Water can tolerate and needs stronger warming and stimulating herbs to clear stagnation. Aggravation of Air, producing fatigue, restlessness or nervousness, needs grounding, and gentle warming with herbs combined with moistening herbs to prevent drying and to nourish and tonify.

Often you will find a mixture of these tendencies in yourself or those you are helping. Here it is best to include herbs affecting each aspect of imbalance; the body will use the energy where it is needed. For example, a Water person may have a headache brought on by constipation or fluid congestion, but may also be experiencing a very stressful situation and be irritable and nervous, indicating involvement of Air imbalance. To clear the headache, choose herbs not only to relieve pain, but others which relax and others to clear the stagnation. Fennel with rosemary, sage or lemon balm, for example, or chamomile and willow bark.

Simples

How many herbs to use? In truth, for short-term, one-off ailments, a single herb can be very effective, provided it is taken strongly and often enough. Such a herb is called a simple.

A good example of simpling is taking echinacea at the first sign of a cold or flu, or eating raw garlic paste (followed by a few sprigs of parsley to cleanse the odour), or drinking copious amounts of elderflower tea. This will either prevent the condition worsening altogether or lighten its course; nothing further needs to be done except to continue with the one herb for a few days extra to thoroughly clear the condition. Try several simples to find the one that best suits you.

Blends

For other ailments that have perhaps happened regularly before or have been around vaguely for a while before they manifest strongly, it is better to use herbs in blends or formulas. The amounts of the different herbs included is important and there are some general guidelines for this.

The greater part of a herbal blend should be given to the herb that most directly affects the condition. For example, in a fever this would be the cooling, antipyretic, blood-purifying herb. This herb can then be reinforced by including the same amount of an extra herb or two with the same main action. Such a herb should also have a secondary action different from that of the main herb but which complements or extends the main action. These three or four herbs are often enough for simple conditions.

If you feel your ailment involves some greater imbalance, weakness or excess, then a more complex blend may be called for. In this case, again choose two or three main but complementary herbs. Then, consider which additional aspect of the body needs support and choose one or two other herbs which extend the action of the blend to this area. For example, in the case of a Water person who has a cold, it would be suggested that laxative and diuretic herbs be added to help clear any residual stagnation in the system. For the Air type, nervine and nourishing herbs would be called for.

Finally, it is a good rule of thumb to include both a circulation-stimulating herb, either mild or strong depending on the individual, which will help to carry the action of the other herbs through to the tissues efficiently, *and* a relaxing herb which will relieve residual tension and allow the tissues to be more receptive to the herbal effects. These can be added at one half the amount of the main herb.

Sample blends

When making herbal blends use equal parts unless otherwise stated. Measuring herbs by weight is most accurate but measuring spoons or handfuls may be acceptable if the herbs are of like texture e.g. all leaves, or roots.

● For headache in an Earth-Water type, associated with sinus congestion, dull ache, sluggish digestion or bowels:
rosemary – stimulating, warming, pain relieving – 2 parts
basil – stimulating, warming, pain relieving, clears congestion in the head – 2 parts
fennel – warming, improves digestion, helps liquify and remove mucous, mildly diuretic so clears excess damp – 1 part
ginger – circulating, warming, antispasmodic – 1/2 part.

● For headache in an Air type, associated with nervous tension or irritability, stress, poor sleep, fatigue, throbbing pain:
skullcap – relaxing, calming, cooling – 1 part
meadowsweet – pain relieving, cooling, soothing – 1 part
vervain – nerve tonic, calming, cooling, decongests liver – 1 part
rosemary – warming, circulating, pain relieving – 1/2 part
ginger – warming, antispasmodic, circulating, grounding – 1/2 part.

Here a small amount of warming herbs are included to guard against an excess of cooling energy in the main herbs.

● For indigestion in a Fire type, associated with acidity, belching, discomfort after eating:
slippery elm powder – demulcent, soothing to mucous membranes, counteracts acidity, grounding – 1 part
meadowsweet – pain relieving, counters acidity, demulcent – 1 part
cumin – cooling, digestive – 1 part
chamomile – relaxing, improves digestion, aromatic – 1 part
peppermint – cooling, improves digestion, pain relieving, stimulating – 1/2 part

Herbal Energetics and Therapeutic Actions

Energy key: Neutral / Warming / Cooling / Drying / Moistening

Humour key: Increases ↑ Decreases ↓ Mixed or Neutral ↔ Air, Fire, Water

HERBS/FOOD	Energy		Carminative	Laxative	Diaphoretic	Diuretic	Expectorant	Demulcent	Astringent	Blood purifying	Nervine	Blood regulating	Tonifying	Vulnerary	HUMOUR
Kitchen herbs															
Allspice	W	D	●		●				●	●		●			F↑ W↓ A↓
Anise	W	D	●		●		●		●	●					F↑ W↓ A↓
Basil	W	D	●		●		●				●	●			F↑ W↓ A↓
Bay	W	D	●		●		●					●			F↑ W↓ A↓
Black pepper	W	D	●				●								F↑ W↓ A↓
Caraway	W		●												F↑ W↓ A↓
Cardamom	W		●				●						●		F↑ W↓ A↑
Cayenne	W	D	●		●		●		●	●		●			F↑ W↓ A↑
Cinnamon	W	D	●		●				●	●					F↑ W↓ A↓
Cloves	W	D	●				●				●				F↑ W↓ A↔
Coriander	C-N		●			●									E, W, A ↔
Cumin	C		●			●									E, W, A ↔
Fennel	C	M	●	●		●	●	●							E, W, A ↔
Fenugreek	W	M	●		●		●	●		●			●		F↑ W↓ A↓
Garlic	W	D	●		●		●			●			●	●	F↑ W↓ A↓
Ginger	W	D	●		●		●				●	●	●		F↑ W↓ A↔
Honey	W	D						●						●	F↑ W↓ A↓
Horseradish	W	D	●		●		●			●			●		F↑ W↓ A↓
Lemon juice	C		●				●		●	●	●		●		F↓ W↔ A↓
Marjoram (oregano)	W		●		●						●				F↑ W↓ A↓
Mung beans	N	M				●				●			●		F↔ W↓ A↓

68

Herbal Energetics and Therapeutic Actions

HERBS/FOOD	ENERGY	Carminative	Laxative	Diaphoretic	Diuretic	Expectorant	Demulcent	Astringent	Blood purifying	Nervine	Blood regulating	Tonifying	Vulnerary	HUMOUR (Increases ↑ / Decreases ↓ / Mixed or Neutral ↔; Air, Fire, Water)
Kitchen herbs cont.														
Mustard	W D	●		●		●			●					F↑ W↓ A↓
Nutmeg	W D	●								●				F↑ W↓ A↓
Oats/oat straw	N		●				●					●		F↓ W↑ A↓
Oil (olive, sesame)	N M		●				●			●		●		F↔ W↑ A↔
Onion	W			●				●	●					F↑ W↓ A↓
Parsley	W	●			●				●					F↑ W↓ A↓
Rosemary	W	●		●		●		●	●	●	●	●		F↑ W↓ A↓
Sage	W D	●		●		●		●	●		●	●		F↑ W↓ A↓
Thyme	W	●		●		●			●	●	●	●		F↑ W↓ A↓
Turmeric	W	●						●	●	●		●	●	F↔ W↓ A↓
Vinegar, Apple cider	C D								●			●		F↑ W↓ A↔
Garden herbs														
Aloe	C M		●				●	●	●				●	Regulates all
Borage	C			●		●	●			●	●			F↑ W↓ A↔
Catnip	C	●		●						●	●			F↓ W↓ A↔
Chamomile	C-N	●		●						●	●			F↓ W↓ A↔
Cornsilk	C				●		●							F↓ W↓ A↔
Dong quai (chinese angelica)	W								●	●		●		Regulates all
Elder flower	C			●	●	●			●					F↓ W↓ A↔

Energy key: Neutral (N), Warming (W), Cooling (C), Drying (D), Moistening (M)

Herbal Energetics and Therapeutic Actions

HERBS/FOOD	ENERGY	Carminative	Laxative	Diaphoretic	Diuretic	Expectorant	Demulcent	Astringent	Blood purifying	Nervine	Blood regulating	Tonifying	Vulnerary	HUMOUR (Increases ↑ Decreases ↓ Mixed or Neutral ↔ Air, Fire, Water)
Garden herbs cont.														
Elecampane	W	●			●	●		●				●		F↑ W↓ A↓
Feverfew	C	●							●			●		F↓ W↓ A↔
Ginseng	W									●	●		●	Tones WFA
Heartsease (pansy)	C			●	●	●	●	●	●	●	●		●	F↓ W↓ A↔
Hibiscus	C M			●			●				●			F↓ W↓ A↑
Hollyhock	C					●			●			●		F↓ W↑ A↓
Honeysuckle	C			●	●				●	●				F↓ W↓ A↑
Hyssop	W D			●		●			●			●		F↑ W↓ A↓
Juniper	W D	●			●				●			●		F↑ W↓ A↓
Lady's mantle	N										●			F↑ W↓ A↓
Lavender	W	●				●			●	●	●			F↓ W↓ A↔
Lemon Balm	C	●		●						●	●			F↓ W↓ A↔
Marigold	C			●			●				●		●	F↓ W↓ A↑
Nasturtium	W	●							●					F↑ W↓ A↑
Peony	C	●		●					●			●	●	F↓ W↓ A↔
Peppermint	C-W								●	●				F↓ W↓ A↔
Periwinkle	N							●	●	●				F↓ W↓ A↔
Skullcap	C								●	●				F↓ W↓ A↔
St Johns wort	C							●	●	●	●	●	●	F↓ W↓ A↔
Vervain	C			●	●					●		●	●	F↓ W↓ A↔
Violet	C					●	●		●		●			F↓ W↓ A↔

Herbal Energetics and Therapeutic Actions

HERBS/FOOD	ENERGY (Neutral/Warming/Cooling/Drying/Moistening)	Carminative	Laxative	Diaphoretic	Diuretic	Expectorant	Demulcent	Astringent	Blood purifying	Nervine	Blood regulating	Tonifying	Vulnerary	HUMOUR (Increases ↑ / Decreases ↓ / Mixed or Neutral ↔ — Air, Fire, Water)
Garden herbs cont.														
Walnut leaf	C							●	●				●	F↑ W↓ A↓
Wood betony	C								●	●		●	●	F↓ W↓ A↔
Wild herbs														
Agrimony	W				●				●	●			●	F↓ W↓ A↔
Barberry	C		●						●		●			F↓ W↓ A↔
Birch twigs	W				●			●	●					F↓ W↓ A↔
Bistort	C				●			●	●			●		F↓ W↓ A↑
Blue flag iris	C		●		●				●		●			F↓ W↓ A↑
Burdock	C			●	●			●	●					F↓ W↓ A↑
Calamus, sweet	W	●							●				●	F↑ W↓ A↓
Chickweed	C				●	●	●		●					F↓ W↓ A↔
Cleavers	C · D				●				●	●				F↓ W↓ A↑
Coltsfoot	C-N					●	●	●						F↓ W↓ A↔
Comfrey	C					●	●	●	●		●	●	●	F↓ W↑ A↑
Couch grass	C				●		●							F↓ W↓ A↔
Dandelion	C	●			●				●			●		F↓ W↓ A↑
Echinacea	C								●			●		F↓ W↓ A↑
Ephedra	W			●		●			●					F↑ W↓ A↑
Eyebright	C							●	●					F↓ W↓ A↑
Flax seed	N · M		●				●		●	●				F↓ W↓ A↑ / Balances all

Herbal Energetics and Therapeutic Actions

HERBS/FOOD	ENERGY (Neutral/Warming/Cooling/Drying/Moistening)		Carminative	Laxative	Diaphoretic	Diuretic	Expectorant	Demulcent	Astringent	Blood purifying	Nervine	Blood regulating	Tonifying	Vulnerary	HUMOUR (Increases ↑ Decreases ↓ Mixed or Neutral ↔ Air, Fire, Water)
Wild herbs cont.															
Gentian, Yellow	C		•												F↓ W↓ A↑
Golden seal	C			•		•			•	•			•	•	F↓ W↓ A↑
Ground ivy	W		•		•				•				•	•	F↑ W↓ A↓
Hawthorn	W		•					•				•	•		F↑ W↔ A↓
Heather	N						•						•		F W A↔
Hops	C		•			•								•	F↓ W↑ A↑
Horsetail	C	D		•		•			•				•		F↑ W↑ A↓
Irish moss	W	M					•	•		•			•		F↑ W↑ A↓
Kelp	C	M				•		•		•			•		F↑ W↑ A↓
Kudzu	C	M	•				•	•					•		F↓ W↑ A↓
Licorice	N	M	•			•	•	•	•	•	•		•	•	W↑ F↓ A↓
Marshmallow	C	M				•	•	•	•		•				F↓ W↑ A↓
Meadowsweet	C	D			•	•	•	•	•		•				F↓ W↓ A↔
Mistletoe leaf	W					•				•	•	•			F↑ W↑ A↓
Motherwort	W		•				•				•		•	•	F↔ W↓ A↑
Mullein	C					•	•	•	•		•		•	•	F↓ W↓ A↑
Nettle	C					•			•	•	•				F↓ W↓ A↑
Passionflower	C										•				F↓ W↓ A↔
Plantain	C					•			•	•				•	F↓ W↓ A↑
Raspberry/ strawberry	C								•	•			•		F↓ W↓ A↑

Herbal Energetics and Therapeutic Actions

HERBS/FOOD	ENERGY (Neutral/Warming/Cooling/Drying/Moistening)	THERAPEUTIC ACTION Carminative	Laxative	Diaphoretic	Diuretic	Expectorant	Demulcent	Astringent	Blood purifying	Nervine	Blood regulating	Tonifying	Vulnerary	HUMOUR (Increases ↑ / Decreases ↓ / Mixed or Neutral ↔ / Air, Fire, Water)
Wild herbs cont.														
Red clover	C						●		●	●		●		F↓ W↓ A↑
Rosehip	N-W	●										●		F↑ W↑ A↑
Self-heal	N-C				●			●	●		●		●	F↓ W↓ A↑
Shepherd's purse	C				●			●	●		●		●	F↓ W↓ A↑
Skullcap	C									●		●		F↓ W↓ A↔
Slippery elm	N (M)					●	●	●				●	●	F↓ W↑ A↓
Squaw vine	C				●			●			●			F↓ W↓ A↑
Uva-ursi (bearberry)	C				●			●						F↓ W↓ A↑
Valerian	W	●			●					●		●		F↑ W↓ A↑
White pine	W (D)			●		●								F↑ W↑ A↑
White willow	C					●		●	●	●				F↓ W↓ A↑
Yarrow	C	●		●	●	●		●		●	●	●	●	F↓ W↑ A↑
Yellow dock	C			●				●	●			●		F↓ W↓ A↑

6

Remedies for Common Ailments

HERBS AND SPECIAL DIETS

COMBINING HERBS WITH special therapeutic diets brings out the best in both herb and diet. Such an approach has long been a part of natural healing in different cultures.

An eliminative, cleansing or reduction diet is one which uses the lighter foods – vegetables and fruits – to promote the eliminations of toxins or congestion which have built up in tissues. This type of diet may adapted for use by any constitutional type when circumstances of excess suggest it, though Water types are especially prone, for example, to retain weight or fluid.

PLEASE NOTE: Cleansing and reduction therapy is only appropriate for those who are basically strong and experiencing excess syndrome, not for those who are deficient or weak.

Cleansing Diet for Acute Ailments

Adopt a light vegetable and fruit diet, taking only freshly pressed juices, or vegetable broths. To the broths and even to the fruit juices, add some ginger, garlic, anise or other warming spice, to balance the cooling effect, especially in winter. At the same time drink herb teas which are diaphoretic, antiseptic and mildly stimulating, such as yarrow, ginger, peppermint, elderflower, thyme, lemon balm. Drink a cup of tea or juice at least every two hours through the day. When coming back to cooked foods, start with puréed soups, then include steamed vegetables, and then baked vegetables before gradually re-introducing normal foods. Continue to use herbs with these foods.

Cleansing Diet for Gradual Reduction

Adopt this diet in conjunction with appropriate herbs when helping the body to rebalance or to reduce excess. It consists simply of avoiding heavy, rich, fried, processed or fast foods as well as animal proteins including eggs, dairy products, salt and stimulants such as sugar, tea and coffee. Replace these with a vegetarian diet based on whole grains, pulses (see especially 'Kitcheree' below), steamed, baked or raw vegetables and fruits, cold-pressed vegetable oils, soya or nut milk and herb teas – combined with your chosen herbs. For maintaining health use it one day per month, for example; or for three days in one week; or for three weeks at the change of the seasons. Many symptoms caused by congestion and excess are relieved once the body has been cleansed.

Potassium broth

Ideal for use during colds, infectious or feverish illnesses, it reduces acidity in the body. To 2 pt (1140 ml) of water add unpeeled, and preferably organic, vegetables: 2 potatoes, 2 carrots, 2 stalks celery, 1 onion and 1 handful of fresh parsley. Cover, bring to the boil and simmer gently until cooked. Season with 1 tsp each of herbs such as fresh or dried ginger, fennel, cayenne or black pepper, and cumin and 3–4 cloves of garlic to taste. Strain the vegetables and serve. For a thicker soup add 1 cup of oats, brown rice or millet that has been soaked overnight then cooked. Purée the whole before serving.

Kitcheree

This herb and food combination comes from India where it is especially used for those convalescing from serious illnesses or those experiencing deficiency or weakness. Also use it for acute ailments and for tonifying the body and at regular intervals to maintain health. It has been called the food of the gods and the ideal food for all types. It provides essential nutrition while being light and eliminative.

1 cup brown or white basmati rice
1/2 cup pre-soaked mung beans or mung dal
1 tbs ghee or cold-pressed vegetable oil
2 pinches turmeric (or more to taste)
1/4 tsp black mustard seeds
1/4 tsp cumin seeds
6 cups water
Fresh coriander, or grated coconut

Wash the rice and beans together. In the pan, warm the ghee or oil on medium heat. Add turmeric, mustard and cumin seeds. When the seeds start to 'crack', add rice, water and beans, stir and cook on low heat, stirring continuously, until the rice and beans are soft (test by squeezing a grain between fingers). Serve with fresh coriander or grated coconut.

HERBS FOR COMMON AILMENTS

The following remedies are suggestions to get you started using herbs. Try them and also feel free to experiment and adapt them according to your experience, using the Table on page 68 and the Materia Medica. Mix the herbs suggested and prepare them according to directions in Hands-on Herbs (page 48). Creating your own blends and discovering what works for you or your family is also enjoyable and satisfying.

Herbs for Digestive Ailments

Acid stomach, indigestion, heartburn

Take one warm cup of any of the following half an hour before eating:

• Tea decoction of a sweet, warming blend: equal parts fennel, licorice, fenugreek, anise, 1/4 part slippery elm or dandelion root.

• Light, minty tea: equal parts meadowsweet, peppermint or spearmint or catnip, 1/2 part rosemary.

• Slice of lemon squeezed in 8 fl oz (227 ml) hot water.

Colic or cramping pains in the intestinal tract

Take the following half an hour before eating or when needed:

• Tea decoction of equal parts ginger, chamomile, catnip.

• For children and babies: equal parts catnip, spearmint or peppermint and fennel. Alternately combine dill with chamomile or lemon balm.

Flatulence

Take one of the following half an hour before eating:

• Tea decoction of equal parts licorice, fennel, fenugreek, ginger.

• Tea decoction of equal parts cardamom, cinnamon or nutmeg, dill and caraway.

Constipation:

• Refer to herbs for laxative action on page 36.

• A typical blend would be raspberry leaves, licorice, slippery elm and fennel. Add ginger, black pepper or cayenne for Water types.

• Taking 3 tbsp of olive oil and 6 tbsp of lemon juice in grapefruit or orange juice first thing in the morning is helpful.

Diarrhoea

• Refer to herbs for carminative and laxative action on pages 35 and 36.

• Fruits high in pectin such as apples and bananas are useful, when grated, mashed and combined with warming, astringent herbs like cinnamon, allspice and nutmeg.

• Tea of equal parts mullein or raspberry, slippery elm, chamomile or catnip, and meadowsweet with 1/4 part ginger or black pepper. Honey is also beneficial.

Haemorrhoids or piles

• Give attention to balancing digestion and bowel elimination.

• Local application of aloe vera gel, or chickweed, calendula or comfrey ointment will soothe and heal local irritations and swellings. In stubborn cases add golden seal or myrrh to the ointment.

Hypoglycaemia

A condition in which an over-secretion of insulin into the blood burns off available blood sugar causing temporary fatigue, coldness, headaches, irritability, palpitations or dizziness. Stress, and hereditary factors may play a part.

• Ensure adequate complex carbohydrate and protein intake through good diet. Brown rice and mung or aduki beans is very beneficial (see Kitcheree).

• Blend equal parts dandelion root, burdock root, licorice root, and skullcap. Take these in tea or powdered form, three times daily.

Irritable bowel and colitis

• A combination of bowel cleansing and tonic herbs with equal the amount of demulcents benefits this tremendously.

• Correct diet and lifestyle.

• Tea or powders in capsules or pills of equal parts licorice root, raspberry, fennel, barberry and rhubarb root. Mix these, then add an equivalent amount of slippery elm or marshmallow root.

Caution: avoid barberry and rhubarb root during pregnancy.

• Take a nervine tea such as chamomile or lemon balm and wood betony, catnip and vervain.

If symptoms persist or if there is any bleeding consult a trained herbalist or medical doctor.

Nausea or vomiting

• Ginger tea from dry or sliced fresh ginger.

• Peppermint tea.

• Juice of a lemon slice in warm water.

• Tea of equal parts cinnamon, cardamom, peppermint or clove or nutmeg.

• Michael Tierra recommends the following combination: 3 parts cinnamon, 1 part each of clove, cardamom and nutmeg. Mix and use 1/4 to 1/2 tsp per cup of water for the brew, or mix powders with honey and eat 1 tsp as needed.

Herbs for Respiratory Ailments

Refer to herbs for carminative, expectorant, diaphoretic and nervine action (Chapter 4, pages 35, 38, 39, 44).

Asthma

• Chronic cases should be referred to a professional herbalist. In mild cases or only occasional and mild crisis, refer to the remedies for colds and flu, and coughs, pages 80, 81.

• During an attack take a hot tea of 1/2 tsp each of ginger and licorice powder. Rub warm sesame oil into the chest.

• Between attacks cleanse the system with a tea of equal parts of thyme, nettle and skullcap. Drink 1 cup of tea 1/2 hour after meals.

- Make a herb pillow with nervine and aromatic herbs, for example lavender and basil.

Ear ache

- Make a herbal oil from garlic, ginger or mullein. Dip a piece of cotton wool in the oil and plug the ear. Renew as needed.

- A poultice made with slippery elm or marshmallow root powder spread around the outside of the ear has proved very effective.

- Take echinacea capsules every 1–2 hours.

Case history
A young mother called me about her 18-month-old daughter who had an ear infection and high temperature. She had just returned from the doctor who had prescribed antibiotics and had recommended she keep her daughter cool to prevent convulsions. The little girl was crying in great pain. I suggested she try the slippery elm poultice and mullein oil in the ear. The mother contrived the poultice and ingeniously smeared some on a towel then put that against her chest and held her daughter to herself. 'Within a very short time you could see the colour of her ear and surrounding skin change from bright red to white. I didn't wash it off and the next day she was a transformed child – energetic, laughing, chattering and is now getting over her infection well.'

Colds and flu

- Adopt a cleansing diet for 1–3 days. Take sweating therapy. Rest.

- Take a tablespoon of garlic oil, or garlic capsules every hour or take two echinacea, thyme or golden seal (singly or combined) capsules every two hours during the day.

- *Trikatu* blend, a combination derived from Ayurvedic tradition, is excellent and also useful for hayfever, sinus congestion and other respiratory allergies. To make *trikatu* (adapted by

Michael Tierra) mix 2 parts anise, 1 part ginger and 1 part black pepper powder, blended with honey to form a paste. Take 1 tsp before meals.

• Tea of equal parts of the following: elderflower and peppermint; thyme and basil; white pine and ginger; yarrow, raspberry and black pepper. Add honey to taste.

Coughs

• Adopt the diet for colds and use the sweating therapy (see page 61), unless weak. To the herbs mentioned for colds add expectorants and demulcent herbs: coltsfoot, comfrey leaves, mullein, hyssop, thyme, elecampane, licorice.

• A cough syrup made of a concentrated tea of thyme mixed with raw sugar and honey has been found effective in stubborn cases and in whooping cough: infuse 1 pt (570 ml) of strong thyme tea and strain. Add 1³/4 lb (0.79 kg) of raw sugar, heat gently in a covered pot, stirring at intervals, until the sugar is dissolved. Skim off the surface accumulation. Cool and store. Take 1 tbs as needed.

External treatments for a cough
• Steam inhalation as described on page 55 is also a valuable treatment for colds and coughs.

• Mustard packs (a poultice of mustard powder and flour or slippery elm) on the chest. Rub chest with olive oil first and remove the pack as the skin begins to redden. Repeat at intervals as needed. Use a mustard or cayenne footbath.

• Chest and upper back massages with blends of 2 drops each of two essential oils in 3 tsp or 15 ml vegetable oil. Choose from eucalyptus, chamomile, thyme, lavender, pine or cypress.

Bronchitis

• Follow the treatment for coughs. Blend trikatu (see colds and flu) with marshmallow root, Irish moss or slippery elm.

Case history
A young teacher came complaining of bronchitis, coughing and fatigue. She had taken a week off work to recover, but wasn't

making much progress. The doctor recommended antibiotics but she wanted to try herbal medicine. I recommended she take echinacea and golden seal capsules every two hours for the first day along with a respiratory formula, also frequently the first day, and a nervine formula. If things improved she was to start taking the herbs (capsuled) three times a day and continue for three weeks. She phoned three days later to say that she was much improved, the cough had mostly subsided, she was able to sleep and was feeling much better.

Respiratory allergies, hayfever

● Treat as for colds. Use *trikatu* blend. Drink hot lemon and honey. Take a powdered blend of ephedra, thyme or pine tops combined with marshmallow root, juniper, chaparral, burdock root, parsley, cayenne or black pepper and golden seal.

● Another helpful combination, from David Frawley and Dr Lad, is turmeric powder warmed in butter with raw sugar; cool, and take one teaspoon of the paste every 1/2 – 1 hour during attacks.

● For red, itchy eyes, bathe eyes in a wash of chamomile, eyebright, raspberry or chrysanthemum-flower tea. Soak a cotton wool pad in the tea and place over the eyes; even a cool black teabag can be used to great effect.

Sinus congestion

● Garlic in capsule form or raw taken regularly clears this condition for many people. Eat a paste with pressed raw garlic mixed with honey. Eat fresh parsley afterwards and a slice of lemon.

● A very strong combination is a blend of equal parts grated horseradish, chopped onion and garlic and a pinch of cayenne. Macerate in apple-cider vinegar for three days. Strain and take 1 tbs 1–3 times a day.

● *Trikatu* blend is effective. Take just before meals.

Sore throat

• Anti-infectious and lymph-clearing herbs are needed, along with soothing demulcents to allay pain. Follow a cleansing diet for one to three days. Rest.

• Gargle with a warm tea of sage or red sage and raspberry leaves with honey. Drink the tea every 1/2 – 1 hour. If possible, take echinacea capsules or tea every hour.

• A good sore throat blend from Farida Sharan is to combine in a blender: 4 tbs honey, 6 tbs lemon juice, 4 tbs apple-cider vinegar, 1/3 clove garlic pressed or 1/4 tsp powder, 1/4 tsp ginger. Process to blend and take as a gargle or syrup. For a drink add hot water up to 8 fl oz (227 ml).

Herbs for Urinary Ailments

Adopt a cleansing diet for a few days, drink lots of pure water.

Cystitis

• Drink a tea of diuretic and urinary cleansing herbs: equal parts dandelion root, nettles, parsley, chickweed, couchgrass, yarrow, cleavers.

• Along with the tea, take anti-infectants such as golden seal and echinacea in capsules. Add to the tea demulcents like marshmallow root, slippery elm. Drink eight or more glasses of pure cranberry, coconut or pomegranate juice daily; and/or eat live, natural yoghourt. Rest.

• If the condition is recurrent and the person feels tired and has a low-grade fever, elimination and tonification treatment should be taken once the acute attack has cleared.

Water retention

The remedies suggested aim to improve kidney excretion to clear any fluid congestion, to promote assimilation of food and elimination of waste, and to clean the blood and lymph and promote circulation. Water types are most easily prone to this pattern, though it is found in all types. Do not confuse it with the deeper oedema based on heart and kidney weakness for which professional treatment is needed.

● Take a digestion-promoting combination given under that section. *Trikatu* blend with meals is excellent.

● Drink teas of mild diuretics which will not over-stimulate the kidneys.

● Diuretic tea combinations: equal parts lemongrass, fennel or coriander or parsley; chickweed, couch grass, cleavers, juniper berries. Water types include a pinch of ginger. Air types should take the tea hot; Fire types take it room temperature; Water types warm with honey.

● Lymph and blood-cleansing herbs can be included in a blend – for example red clover, chaparral, burdock, echinacea – along with circulatory stimulants such as ginger, cayenne and black pepper.

Urinary stones

These can be dissolved with herbal treatment.

● A typical blend would include chickweed, cleavers, juniper berries, parsley root, dandelion, golden seal with marshmallow root to protect against pain and irritation. Take this as a tea, 1 cup three times a day for three weeks.

● In an acute crisis of urinary colic Farida Sharan uses a strong decoction of 2 oz (56 g) hydrangea root soaked thoroughly then simmered in 32 fl oz (910 ml) pure apple juice for 20 minutes. Drink 2 fl oz (50 ml) every hour when awake. Repeat as needed. Adopt a cleansing diet or kitcheree diet for one week.

Herbs for Skin Ailments

Skin ailments usually indicate imbalances deeper in the system which the body is trying to resolve by elimination through the skin. Topical remedies must be combined with systemic treatment according to constitutional type.

Acne

Contributing factors are poor diet (junk foods like chocolate, fried foods, coffee, tea, refined flour and sugar products), stress, liver congestion, and hormonal imbalance.

• Have daily steam facials with cleansing herbs such as sage, eucalyptus, rosemary and thyme.

• Apply soothing ointments of calendula or comfrey; antiseptic and cleansing aloe vera gel; a paste made from turmeric and slippery elm mixed with a little water.

• Internally, take a tea of 1–3 of the following blood-purifying and kidney and liver cleansing herbs: alfalfa, echinacea, red clover, burdock, dandelion, licorice, nettle, sassafras, yarrow, yellow dock, plantain and cleavers. Drink 1 cup, 3 times a day.

• Avoid foods that stimulate the Fire humour: fried foods, greasy and rich foods, tomatoes and hot spices.

• Take a hormone blend such as the one suggested under Reproductive Ailments, pages 95–6.

Athlete's foot

• Go barefoot whenever possible; wear only cotton socks. Take daily foot baths in tea of rosemary and thyme with 2 tbs lemon juice or cider vinegar.

• Massage feet with essential oils of lemon, ti-tree, eucalyptus, lavender, thyme or rosemary – up to four drops diluted in about 3 tsp or 15 ml of carrier vegetable oil.

• Internally, take garlic or echinacea capsules.

Allergies, skin rashes, insect bites, stings

• Apply a slippery elm or marshmallow root poultice or fomentation combined with drinking a tea of chamomile, calendula, or plantain. Also bathe the area with these herb teas and take a herb tea bath.

• Apply aloe vera gel; marigold, comfrey or chickweed ointment.

Dandruff

• Correct the diet, cutting out junk and processed foods. Try a vitamin and mineral supplement or take kelp tablets. Check that your shampoo is mild and natural.

• After shampooing, rinse with a tea made with rosemary, nettles, nasturtium combined with half the amount of apple-cider vinegar. When possible massage scalp with warm olive oil combined with 2 drops of rosemary essential oil.

• Daily, drink nettle and sage or rosemary tea to cleanse the blood and improve circulation.

Eczema

Treatment for this condition needs to be discussed with a professional herbalist but for temporary relief, for mild conditions or when it first appears try the following.

• Apply oil of evening primrose.

• Bathe the area with tea of marigold, comfrey leaves, chamomile, marshmallow root.

• Macerate in oil: lavender, chamomile, calendula, comfrey or marshmallow leaves and apply twice daily.

• An ointment made with balm of Gilead buds is very effective.

• Internally, take teas of blood-purifying, heat-releasing herbs such as burdock root, red clover, yarrow, marshmallow root, calendula, elderflower, nettle or chamomile; and nervine teas to allay anxiety and stress: chamomile, skullcap, lemon balm, catnip, vervain or wood betony.

Eye inflammations, styes

• Make a tea with slippery elm or marshmallow root and eyebright, calendula, borage, elderflower, honeysuckle flower, fennel powder or chamomile. Strain and cool. Soak a cotton wool ball in the tea and apply to the eyelid and area around eye; give an eyewash using an eyecup.

• Take echinacea capsules for a few days to boost the immune system.

Insect repellants

● Massage into the skin a herbal oil of lavender, thyme, marjoram, basil, citrus lemon peel, rose geranium, bay leaves or even garlic. Use essential oil of citronella or the above herbs diluted into a carrier oil.

Psoriasis

● Seek help from a qualified herbalist but for relief try bathing the area in kelp or other seaweeds and taking kelp tablets.

● Apply poultices or herb teas of cooling, demulcent herbs such as slippery elm, marshmallow root, comfrey, calendula. Drink a blood-purifying tea blend (see p.37).

● Avoid all heating spices and greasy or fried foods, even meat.

Wounds, infections, boils, abrasions

● Apply aloe vera gel or a poultice or ointment of plantain, comfrey, marigold, St John's wort, yarrow, slippery elm, lemon balm, chamomile, thyme or self-heal.

● When in the wild make an emergency poultice by chewing the leaves of one of these or other recognized wound herbs, and place them on the wound.

● Honey is another antiseptic first aid remedy.

Burns

● Aloe vera gel is excellent.

● Apply comfrey or marigold ointment.

● An excellent combination for severe burns, from Dr Christopher: in a blender mix equal parts wheat-germ oil and honey (the amount judged according to the area to be covered).

Gradually add chopped fresh or dry (powdered) comfrey leaves to form a paste. Apply cool and leave on the burn WITHOUT disturbing it until the skin underneath has healed. Remoisten at intervals with comfrey and chickweed tea. This also relieves itching. Avoid exposure of new skin to sunlight for one year.

Herbs for Circulatory and Lymphatic Ailments

Chilblains

● Take tepid footbaths with 2 tbs ginger, mustard or cayenne powder. Apply crushed onion.

● Rub the area with comfrey, or calendula ointment. Avoid the temptation to immediately apply heat as this will only worsen the situation with sudden dilation. Gentle re-warming is called for.

● To strengthen the circulation and capillaries, drink a daily tea of ginger, marjoram, cloves, cumin, thyme, hawthorn berries, nettle or buckwheat. Take garlic capsules daily.

Swollen glands

● Tea or powders in capsules or pills of lymph-clearing herbs: equal parts of mullein, echinacea, garlic, dandelion root and red clover.

● Poke root is a specific, but must not be used during pregnancy.

● Apply a poultice of astringents such as oak bark, walnut leaves, or mullein with fennel, fenugreek, marshmallow root or slippery elm powders over the area.

Swollen ankles or knees

● Lightly apply essential oil blends of cypress, cedarwood or fennel, diluted in vegetable oil.

● Apply a salt pack: warm the salt in the oven, enough to cover the area to 1/4 in (6 mm); wrap it in a tea-towel and apply over the area. Leave for an hour or overnight.

● Take a diuretic tea blend to reduce excess damp such as ginger with dandelion, burdock, cleavers and horsetail.

General coldness

● Include ginger or black pepper, and cardamom in your daily drinks and foods. Massage sesame oil into the body two or three times a week and on the soles of the feet at bedtime.

Excess weight

• Activate elimination, make dietary changes and exercise regularly. Herbs can greatly help this condition by activating the eliminative channels and supporting the body while diet is reduced.

• A typical blend would be equal parts kelp, parsley leaves or root, chickweed, burdock, fennel, cayenne and ginger. Take a tea or 2 capsules of powder 3 times daily.

• Take *trikatu* blend with meals.

• Take the bowel cleansing tonic given for constipation (p.77). Adopt a diet rich in fresh vegetables, whole grains, fruits and avoid flour products, processed foods, eggs, cheese and milk, meat, salt and sugar for three weeks. Rest one week and repeat as needed.

Herbs for Muscles and Joints

Arthritis

This is often a condition of excess damp and toxicity accumulating in the fluid and tissues around the joints producing stiffness, low-grade inflammation and consequent soreness. There may be an acute phase with greater inflammation, swelling, heat and redness.

• Local applications: warm stiff, sore joints with fresh ginger juice: grate some root and squeeze the juice into some vegetable oil, rub into the area. Apply the Kloss liniment described on page 57. Use two handfuls of Epsom salts in the bath.

• Sweating therapy is especially indicated for arthritis in Fire and Water types. Air types may use it if they are strong. Drink diaphoretic teas before entering a steam bath. Cool down at intervals and at the end.

• Internally take blood purifying and circulation herbs to warm and disperse. For example, equal parts alfalfa, red clover, mullein, skullcap, chickweed or nettles, parsley and hibiscus. Take 1 cup 2–3 times a day. The tea may need to be taken for about three months, alternating the herbs in the blend every week.

● When there is acute pain, inflammation, redness and swelling, apply a cooling poultice of marshmallow root.

Back pain

While back pain may be structural in origin and massage, osteopathy or chiropractic can help, it can also be due to a weakening or stress of kidney function.

● Use the remedies for sciatica and also take a kidney tonifying blend such as the following: Tea or decoction: 1 part each of marshmallow root, parsley root or leaf, cleavers, horsetail and juniper berries with 1/4 part ginger.

Strain or sprain

● Follow this RICE procedure when the injury occurs:
 1. Rest
 2. Apply cold in the form of Ice or frozen peas
 3. Apply a Compression bandage
 4. Elevate the injury so blood flows toward the heart.

● Additionally, apply the Kloss liniment (see page 57) or a fomentation, oil or poultice of yarrow, comfrey or St John's wort tea mixed with blood moving herbs such as ginger or dong quai. A comfrey poultice will also help. Drink a tea of comfrey leaf, St John's wort leaves and walnut leaves if available. (Commercially produced homeopathic remedies such as Arnica 6, and Bach Flower Star of Bethlehem or Rescue Remedy may be taken.)

● In contrast to the cold treatment recommended above, Chinese medicine recommends applying heat. Heat is said to promote blood circulation, so clearing swelling, pain and stasis sooner.

Sciatica

This is pain along the sciatic nerve. The nerve emerges from the sacrum to ennervate the legs and feet. Pain is often due to disc prolapse, especially at the fifth lumbar vertebra, or to structural or postural imbalance affecting the vertebrae, involving the muscles of the buttocks, sacrum and pelvis. A remedial massage therapist, chiropractor or osteopath should be consulted; specific exercises may be given to improve the situation. The following herbal remedies have also proved helpful to many people as poor diet and lack of exercise can cause blood and lymph stagnation which can accumulate in the tissues in this area and also provoke or contribute to the pain.

• Externally: apply a 2 tsp ginger and 1 tsp turmeric paste, warm, to the area. St John's wort oil or the Kloss liniment may be rubbed into the area for temporary relief. Use an essential oil massage blend choosing three of the following: lavender, rosemary, chamomile, peppermint, black pepper, eucalyptus or wintergreen.

• Baths with these herbs as teas are also good.

• Internally: drink willow bark, nettle or chamomile tea. Take St John's wort tincture.

Herbs for Nervous Ailments

Refer to nervine action herbs (page 44).

Anxiety

• Take a tea of skullcap, borage, chamomile, and/or lemon balm.

• Basil tea and sandalwood essential oil used as a massage rub or room scent promote a calm but alert mind.

Depression

• Borage tea conveys courage. Lemon balm is traditionally good for melancholia, that feeling of dejection and withdrawal from the world. Lemon balm tea from fresh leaves is best; if this is not possible use 4 drops essential oil of melissa in a bath or footbath daily. Balm is both relaxing to the nerves and uplifting to the spirits as are most of the aromatic herbs – basil, rosemary, lavender and many others.

• According to Rudolph Weiss, St John's wort is used by European herbalists to treat depression: take as a tea twice a day. It has a cumulative effect so may need to be taken for several weeks before a change is noticed. Adding ginger to a blend will help circulate energy and break up stagnation. Herbs used regularly can be effective.

• Refer to the section on reproductive ailments, page 93.

Headaches

The head can be a focal point for the expression of imbalances elsewhere, for example stomach upsets, constipation, excess mucous congesting the sinuses, excess water or lymph congestion, and liver congestion. Issues of stress or nervous tension can cause headaches. Such background causes should be given treatment by referring to the appropriate section. Diet may be a factor so food therapy may be useful.

• Internally, take a tea of 1–3 of the following: meadowsweet, willow bark, poplar bark, lime flowers, peppermint, chamomile, skullcap, rosemary, ginger, wood betony, valerian, basil, lemon balm, passion flower or sage.

• A tea of cumin and coriander is also helpful for headaches based on liver congestion.

• For occipital headaches (at the back of the head) take a colon-cleansing blend such as flax or senna at bedtime with warm milk.

• Meadowsweet, willow bark, and poplar bark all contain salicylic acid, the active ingredient in aspirin, and will relieve pain.

• Externally apply a ginger paste (powdered ginger mixed with a little turmeric and water) to the forehead and sinuses for sinus headaches and behind the ears for occipital headaches.

Fatigue and stress

• Take a nervine tea of 1–3 of the following: skullcap, wood betony, chamomile, catnip, lemon balm, rosemary or vervain.

• Tonify the glandular system with the hormone blend given for reproductive ailments, adding ginseng.

• Herbs to build the quality of the blood may also be beneficial: take a daily tea, equal parts of 1–3 of the following: nettles, yarrow, burdock, yellow dock, alfalfa, dong quai or comfrey leaves.

Insomnia

• During the afternoon and early evening drink a tea of 1–3 of the following: valerian, catnip, lemon balm, lime flowers, hops, wood betony, passionflower, skullcap or chamomile. Continue this for several days even after sound sleep returns.

• Make a herbal pillow with the following herbs: hops, lavender, passionflower, skullcap and valerian. Place it in your pillowcase.

• Apply a few drops of lavender or other relaxant essential oil (melissa, ylang ylang, frankincense, sandalwood, marjoram) on a handkerchief attached to the pillow.

Withdrawal symptoms

For those withdrawing from drugs – whether cigarettes, alcohol, narcotics, or tranquillizers – nervine herbs offer support and relieve symptoms. The following is a blend which is used by drug detoxification centres such as the Lincoln Clinic in New York City and the Gateway Centre in London.

• Equal parts chamomile, yarrow, hops, skullcap, catnip and peppermint. Take one cup of tea every hour when symptoms are acute along with frequent hot baths.

Herbs for Female Reproductive Ailments

Herbs have much help to offer in creating and maintaining balance: some are used for their cleansing and tonifying action on the organs, blood and lymph; others relax and relieve cramp and pain. There are herbs that contain plant hormones which are precursors to human hormones: their molecular structure is very similar and the body can use components of them to augment its hormone production. Cleansing and balancing on the physical level will be reflected in feelings of well-being throughout the body.

Depression

See Herbs for Nervous Ailments and Hormonal changes.

Excessive bleeding

Energetically, this is considered a condition of excess heat in the blood and causes may include an excess of warming herbs and beverages, hot spices, sour foods, salt, alcohol, and at a more subtle level hot emotions such as anger, or resentment. Fire types are perhaps a little more prone to this. However, excessive bleeding can also be due to other factors such as incomplete (and unknown) miscarriage, cervical erosion, endometriosis, polyps and tumours, so professional advice should always be consulted.

● For relief of minor discomfort of a heavy period take blood cleansing and cooling herbs such as tea of red clover, yarrow, and peppermint, along with astringents such as raspberry leaves and shepherd's purse.

● Blood regulators such as dong quai are also important, as are hormone balancers. Adopt a cleansing diet for three weeks.

Irregular periods

● Take a tea of 1 to 3 of the following herbs: yarrow, motherwort, raspberry, lemon balm, lady's mantle, chamomile, thyme and peppermint plus blood regulators like dong quai.

Hot flushes

● Take a tea of rosemary, sage and lemon balm or peppermint. Drink 1 cup three times a day. Take a hormone combination, such as the one suggested below, and a blood purifying blend.

Period pain

If severe and prolonged, this can indicate a more serious condition so consult a trained practitioner or doctor.

• Use warming, antispasmodic, and blood regulating herbs which relieve cramp such as cramp bark, turmeric, fennel, angelica, dong quai, wild yam, ginger and chamomile.

• Agnus castus is especially helpful as it increases the level of progesterone, a hormone that prevents uterine contractions. Drink a tea combining it with raspberry and the antispasmodic herbs for a week before the onset of the period.

• Taking a hormone combination such as the one for pre-menstrual tension is also advised. Take two capsules three times a day.

Pre-menstrual tension

Symptoms of bloating, sore breasts, headaches and irritability around the start of the period can be related to lymph or blood stagnation and general congestion.

• Take a herb tea to clear excess water (diuretic), cleanse the blood and bowels (liver cleansing and laxative), and support the reproductive organs with a daily tea of raspberry leaves, motherwort, and/or squaw vine. Include a warming, circulating herb such as ginger.

• For temporary relief of headache take a nervine such as rosemary, willow bark or skullcap.

Hormonal changes

The sexual turning points of life, from puberty to the menopause, can be stressful for the body as they carry us from one phase of life into another. We can give our health support by natural means even if we do not experience any unpleasant symptoms at these times, so building our health for the future. If we experience symptoms, we need to deal with them promptly as imbalances not resolved at the time may manifest themselves again later in life.

At these times the body is undergoing immense changes which can alter its normal balance. Using the following hormone blend periodically through these years can minimize any negative effects and leave the body stronger. Take it for three weeks at a time.

• *Hormone Blend*: a basic combination to use for good hormone function at the life-changes and for menstrual problems is equal parts kelp, dong quai, ginseng, sarsaparilla, agnus castus, wild yam, licorice, false unicorn, fennel, black cohosh. Combine with a smaller amount of ginger and a nervine such as chamomile or vervain. Take in capsule, tea or decoction form three times daily for three weeks. Repeat as needed. For period problems take three times a day for one week before the period every month for at least three months.

Pregnancy and childbirth

Herbs can be very helpful to counteract the minor discomforts of pregnancy and to strengthen the muscles for childbirth. Pregnancy is not the time to embark on a cleansing programme, though it is a good idea to do so before conception.

● For nausea, take a pinch of ginger in weak tea or hot water with a slice of lemon.

● Drink raspberry leaf tea regularly throughout pregnancy. In the last six weeks begin to tone the muscles with a tea of raspberry leaves, squaw vine, or motherwort.

● Prepare the vaginal area by massaging wheat-germ oil (1–2 tsp) daily into the perineum and vulva.

● During childbirth, essential oils such as jasmine, lavender, chamomile and clary sage may be used in massage and as room scents to comfort the mother.

● To promote lactation drink fennel, dill or basil tea. For engorged breasts apply a sage compress. Apply calendula or comfrey ointment to sore nipples.

● To calm a restless baby, the nursing mother can drink chamomile or other nervine teas. The effects will be conveyed to the baby through the milk. An older infant may be bathed in a bath to which chamomile tea is added, or given a teaspoon of chamomile tea before sleep.

● Herbs to be avoided during pregnancy include golden seal, poke root, dong quai, angelica, barberry, hyssop, senna, turkey rhubarb, rue and vervain. The following culinary herbs should be used with some caution, especially in the first trimester; they are safe for occasional or short-term use and in cooking, but the worry is that with prolonged or concentrated use their stimulating properties may provoke a miscarriage or premature labour in a, perhaps unknown, susceptible state: fennel, fenugreek, cayenne, garlic, thyme, sage, marjoram, juniper, cinnamon, parsley and peppermint. On the other hand, they may be taken at the end of term to help prepare for labour.

Menopause

• Take the hormone blend and combine with a nervine tea. See also Hot Flushes, page 94.

• Scanty flow: take a tea or powders in capsules of warming, blood moving, emmenagogue (promoting menstrual discharge) herbs such as dong quai, fennel, vervain, yarrow along with a reproductive tonic such as raspberry or motherwort.

Vaginal discharge

In simple cases this is usually due to an imbalance in the acidity of the area, often brought on by antibiotics, a diet too high in sugar, processed and acid forming foods, or to thrush, a fungal infection. Correct the diet.

• To relieve itching, apply calendula or chickweed ointment, or simply olive or wheatgerm oil. Vulval itching is an important symptom in diabetes so repeated or prolonged itching suggests a consultation with a doctor would be in order.

• Douche with yoghourt mixed with the same amount of water, or with yellow dock tea.

• Vaginal pessaries with essential oil of ti-tree and lavender are now available and may be used.

• Take herbal antibiotics such as echinacea, golden seal and chaparral in tea or capsule form.

• A home-made bolus of slippery elm powder, yellow dock root and golden seal (equal parts) can also be effective: mix with melted coconut oil and 1 drop ti-tree essential oil to form a dough, shape into a 1 inch, finger-size pessary and insert into vagina, following with a cut-off tampon to hold it in place. Leave overnight and douche in the morning. Repeat three nights. If the problem persists, consult qualified help.

Herbs for Male Ailments

Prostate swelling

This condition appears in some men as they pass into their middle and later years. In the beginning stages and in mild cases, there is pain or burning on urination due to the swelling of the gland and consequent pressure on the urethra.

● Take the following hormone combination in tea or powdered, capsule form: juniper berries, couchgrass, horsetail and hydrangea root. Take echinacea and/or golden seal.

Puberty and/or stress

● Men can also benefit from the recommended hormone combination during puberty, pages 95–6, in middle and older age and whenever affected by a time of stress. It strengthens the glandular function in both sexes and enhances vitality and vigor.

Herbs for Fevers and Infections

Fevers and infections, when temporary, are due to a combination of excess Fire (heat-toxins and pathogens) or Water (phlegm and mucous) in the blood or lymph which allow pathogens to thrive in this milieu. The body raises its temperature to burn off the excess and destroy the bacteria or virus.

● Choose blood purifying, diaphoretic and antibiotic herbs. Herbs to use in teas or capsules include golden seal, echinacea, chaparral, burdock, yarrow, garlic, thyme and sage.

● If there is no high blood pressure or signs of deficiency and weakness, sweating therapy is very useful.

● For local external skin infections or boils, take the recommended herbs internally and also apply a poultice of plantain, slippery elm, marshmallow root, and golden seal or thyme.
If fevers recur often, consult a qualified herbalist or doctor.

Herbs for First Aid

Keep some herbs and preparations on hand for emergencies, while travelling and for the most common complaints.

• Chickweed, comfrey or calendula ointment for wounds and sores.

• Cayenne tincture for shock, bleeding and fainting.

• Herbal liniment: Kloss' liniment is excellent, or one from equal parts juniper, basil and ginger. Use for wounds, muscular aches and sprains.

Herb tea blends can be used for many common ailments.

• For colds and flu: elderflower and peppermint; chamomile and lemon balm.

• For pain relief: willow bark and rosemary; meadowsweet and ginger.

• For 'stomach bug' (short-term gastroenteritis): ginger, slippery elm or licorice, and cinnamon.

• For soothing and sleep: catnip, hops, chamomile, wood betony, vervain or lime flowers.

• For cramps: catnip, ginger and fennel.

• For nausea: ginger and peppermint.

• Herbal antibiotics: equal parts echinacea and golden seal powders in capsules.

7

Herbs on Hand

THERE IS A saying among herbalists: 'It is better to know a few herbs well than a smattering of many'. Since one herb can serve successfully in several conditions because of its multiple therapeutic effects, it is possible to have on hand relatively few herbs and yet be able to treat a wide variety of complaints.

BASIC MATERIA MEDICA

Materia medica means the materials of medicine – a listing of herbs with a description of their characteristics, parts used and properties. The list presented here is necessarily limited but tries to include herbs which are easy to find commercially, in gardens or in the wild, as well as four extremely useful oriental herbs. Please refer to The Herb Chart and the books listed in Further Reading for more information on these and other herbs.

ALOE VERA
Aloe vera (A. barbadensis)

Parts used: flesh of leaf stems.
Properties: blood purifier, antiseptic, healing, antipyretic, purgative, laxative.

Energy: cooling, moistening. Reduces Fire, clears stagnant water, calms Air.

Caution: do not use aloe internally in presence of internal bleeding or heavy menstruation.

A plant that deserves a place in every garden or home. In colder climates it thrives as a houseplant. It is the first aid plant *par excellence*: one only has to pinch off a bit of the fleshy leaves and peel back the outer skin to obtain the cooling antiseptic and healing properties of the clear gel. Use for acne, skin complaints, burns and wounds. Take internally, 1tsp diluted with water, for blood cleansing and as a bowel cleanser.

BASIL
Ocimum basilicum

Parts used: leaves, flowering stem.

Properties: energy stimulant, respiratory decongestant, carminative, diaphoretic, nervine. Uplifts and clears the mind and head.

Energy: warming, clearing, dispersing; Increases Fire, reduces excess Water, calms Air.

Caution: avoid prolonged concentrated use during first trimester of pregnancy. Safe for occasional tea, culinary and short-term uses.

The Indian species of basil holds a high place in Ayurvedic medicine. It is planted around the doors of houses for its purifying effect both on the physical and the emotional and mental levels. All basils reduce excess mucous, and improve digestion. They have a refreshing, uplifting and purifying quality. They are easy to grow annuals that should be used regularly in cooking as well as for medicine.

BAYBERRY
Myrica pennsylvanica

Part used: bark.

Properties: stimulant, aromatic. Clears excess mucous (Water), diaphoretic, expectorant, astringent.

Energy: warming, stimulating, increases Fire, reduces excess Water, calms Air.

Bayberry is a North American herb highly valued by the Thomsonians and Eclectics and many frontier or rural Americans for its stimulating properties. Together with pine, cloves, ginger and cayenne it formed the famous Composition Powder used to mobilize the body's energy to fight off infections and fevers. Bayberry is most used today for conditions of excess mucous such as colds and sinus congestion, even mucous in the intestines and bowel inflammation.

BURDOCK
Arctium lappa

Parts used: root.
Properties: blood purifier, tonic, diuretic, diaphoretic, astringent.
Energy: cool, drying. Reduces Fire, reduces excess Water, increases Air mildly.

Burdock is one of those valuable weeds of fields and waysides. It cleanses the blood through its action on both the liver and the kidneys. Overburdened blood is a major factor behind arthritis, fevers, infections and skin conditions such as boils and sores. Being a starchy root it also supplies nutrition and builds strong blood with its iron content. Yellow dock, although not related botanically, has similar properties.

CALAMUS, SWEET
Acorus calamus

Part used: root.
Properties: nutritive tonic, nervine and brain tonic, digestive aid, clears mucous. Circulating and invigorating.

Energy: warming, calming. Reduces excess Water. Calms and strengthens Air. Mildly increases Fire.
Caution: use this herb only for short terms.

Sweet calamus grows naturally near ponds and waterways. It holds a high place in Ayurvedic medicine as being purifying to the body and the mind and promoting longevity with its rejuvenating qualities. It tonifies digestion, thereby clearing the blood and lymph, and the nerves. Like comfrey it is a starchy root with nutritive qualities. Used externally as a locally applied paste it calms headaches and pain. In the US it is currently listed as not recommended by the Food and Drugs Administration (FDA) for internal use, though it is used thus routinely in India and in the UK.

CATNIP
Nepeta cataria

Parts used: leaves, flowering stem.
Properties: nervine, reduces fever, gently carminative, diaphoretic, stomachic.
Energy: cooling and balancing.

Catnip is especially good for children and the elderly for its action is gently stimulating and clearing while still being effective. It is best combined with fennel for digestive and calming effects.

CAYENNE
Capsicum annuum var. annuum

Parts used: fruit.
Properties: heating, stimulating, blood regulator/haemostatic, diaphoretic, anti-infectious, astringent, carminative, antispasmodic.
Energy: hot, stimulating. Increases Fire but can also disperse excess heat.

Caution: avoid concentrated prolonged use in pregnancy, hypertension and peptic ulcers.

Cayenne is certainly a herb to have on hand for emergencies. It counters shock and can arrest bleeding by its astringency and ability to quickly penetrate tissue and to normalize blood flow – that is to channel its concentration away from the site, whether internal or external. (See Herbs for First Aid.) Its warmth improves circulation to stiff joints, easing them. It benefits digestion and is powerful for clearing excess mucous from the stomach. Dr Christopher used it for stomach ulcers. It normalizes both high and low blood pressure. Cayenne is often an ingredient in formulas for its ability to carry the other herbs quickly where they are needed. It can be taken on a daily basis of 1/4–1 tsp taken at breakfast mixed with juice, water or yoghourt. Chillies are used similarly.

CHAMOMILE
Chamaemelum nobile and *Matricaria recutita*

Parts used: flowering heads.
Properties: carminative, aromatic, diaphoretic, nervine. Roman Chamomile (*Chamaemelum nobile*) is more anti-inflammatory, German chamomile (*Matricaria recutita*) is more antispasmodic.
Energy: cooling, calming. Reduces excess Water, cools Fire, stabilizes Air.

For those who enjoy its soft apple-like flavour, chamomile is a good all-purpose remedy. It helps induce calmness and sound sleep. It clears digestive upsets. It helps clear mucous build-up, so can be used for colds, fever and flu. It is perhaps ideal for Fire types who, through stress, anger and overwork get digestive upsets, sleep poorly or come down with a bad cold. The flavour is often attractive to children making it an excellent choice when treating them for complaints such as poor sleep, upset stomach or colds.

CHAPARRAL
Larrea divaricata

Parts used: leaves and stems.
Properties: blood and lymph purifier, antibiotic, diuretic, expectorant.
Energy: cooling, stimulating. Reduces excess Fire.
Caution: should only be used under professional direction.

Chaparral is a plant from the western United States. It is excellent as a natural antibiotic, often combined with echinacea and golden seal. It is used for colds, flu and fever or inflammation because it cleanses the causative factors in the blood and lymph. Like all herbal antibiotics, while doing its job it strengthens rather than depletes the body's own immune system. Recent reports of possible toxicity have placed the safety of Chaparral for self-medication in some doubt. Until the issue is resolved, avoid using this herb.

CHICKWEED
Stellaria media

Parts used: leaves and flowering stems.
Properties: demulcent, astringent, diuretic, vulnerary.
Energy: cooling, reduces excess Water, cools Fire, mildly increases Air.

Although considered an invasive weed, this plant should be allowed a corner in every garden. It can be eaten as a pot-herb in salads. It is excellent as a mild diuretic, stimulating to the kidneys, reducing weight and water. Used in ointments or as a bath tea, it is beneficial for wounds and skin complaints such as itching, redness and inflammation.

CLEAVERS
Galium aparine

Parts used: leaves and flowering stems.
Properties: diuretic, blood purifying, laxative.

Energy: cooling, drying. Reduces Water, cools Fire, mildly increases Air.

Cleavers are those prolific garden weeds that have a strange dry, sticky texture so that they will cling when pressed against the body. Children enjoy playing with them for this reason. This herb has similar uses to chickweed but is a stronger diuretic. As well as benefiting skin problems and fevers, it finds a place in weight-reduction formulas and to treat oedema and clear kidney stones.

CLOVE
Eugenia caryophyllus

Parts used: flowering bud.
Properties: nervine – anaesthetic, analgesic – aromatic, digestive and circulatory stimulant, carminative, expectorant.
Energy: warming, stimulating. Reduces excess water (mucous, damp), increases Fire, calms Air.

Cloves are used mainly to improve digestive upsets and to clear excess mucous in the lungs, for example in asthma, coughs or colds. As warming carminatives they improve digestion and assimilation of foods and can so raise energy levels and lower blood pressure. Their nervine-analgesic, even numbing, properties provide relief for toothaches and other pain.

COLTSFOOT
Tussilago farfara

Parts used: leaves, flowers.
Properties: demulcent, expectorant, astringent.
Energy: cooling, dispersing.

Coltsfoot's name describes the hoof-like shape of its leaves. It grows easily in damp waste places and will grow quickly in the

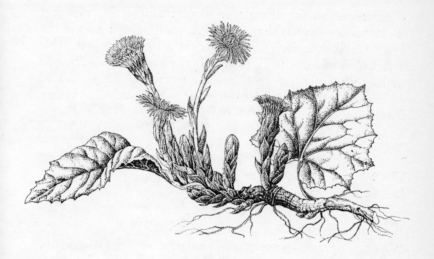

Figure 3   Coltsfoot

garden, so plant it in a container or out-of-the-way spot. It appears very early in spring and is very interesting visually for the dandelion-like flowers come before the leaves. Coltsfoot is a tried and true remedy for coughs, helping to liquify mucous, cool irritated passages and expel the phlegm. It will also relieve diarrhoea due to its astringent action. Crushed leaves make a good poultice for stings and bites.

COMFREY
Symphytum officinalis

Parts used: leaves and flowers. Root under direction of herbalist.
Properties: tonic, demulcent, blood regulator – arrests bleeding and builds blood; vulnerary (tissue healing). Especially good for respiratory system, weakness and anaemia, muscular system.
Energy: cooling, nutritive tonic. Strengthens Water essence and vital fluids. Cools Fire.

There has been a lot of controversy over comfrey, as claims have been made, based on flawed research, that it is carcinogenic. Yet comfrey is one of those invaluable herbs. It can be used as an organic feed for garden plants when used as a green manure or after being composted. Its leaves can be eaten as a spring pot-herb vegetable. As medicine it especially benefits the lungs, is soothing to coughs and bronchial inflammation. In wasting diseases the starchy root is used as a nutritive tonic and renewer of tissue. It can stop bleeding and heal external and internal tissues. So it is beneficial where bleeding occurs from ulcers, lungs, kidneys or bowels. Comfrey is a tremendous healer of minor or severe burns and wounds, soothing the trauma and promoting growth of new, healthy tissue.

CRAMP BARK
Viburnum opulus

Parts used: inner bark of limbs.
Properties: antispasmodic, nervine, astringent.
Energy: warming, relaxing. Calms Air.

Cramp bark and its relative Black haw (*Viburnum prunifolium*) are valued for their effects on menstrual cramps, especially when combined with ginger. The warmth circulates energy in the pelvic region, relieving blood congestion; the antispasmodic action relaxes excessive uterine contractions; the astringency tones the tissues. Its nervine action is general and also benefits heart palpitations and asthma.

CUMIN
Cuminum cyminum

Parts used: seeds.
Properties: carminative, digestive aid, antispasmodic, stimulant, alterative.
Energy: warming and cooling. Reduces excess Fire and Water. Calms Air.

Cumin is one of the culinary spices which is useful for many medicinal purposes. It alleviates gas and indigestion, colic and diarrhoea. Fire types especially should use it regularly and especially with heating foods like tomatoes or hot spices as it counteracts their heating effects. It will improve the assimilation of foods and therefore can be used to treat weakness and deficiency.

DANDELION
Taraxacum officinalis

Parts used: leaves and root.
Properties: diuretic, blood purifier, liver tonic, stomachic, nutritive.
Energy: cooling. Reduces excess Water (damp), cools Fire, stabilizes Air.

Dandelion is a very important herb, finding a place in the treatment of both acute and chronic illnesses. Herbalists use it as part of treatment for diabetes, kidney and gall bladder obstructions, heart disease, and liver disease such as hepatitis. Both the leaves and the root are nutritive, providing valuable minerals; the root is stronger and preferred for medicinal use, though the leaves are also valuable. It is an excellent blood purifier through its action both on the liver and the kidneys, as its French name *pis en lit* (wet the bed) tells us. It can be used for acute stomach aches in the form of a decoction and to help reduce excess weight. Regular use from time to time keeps the internal organs clear and healthy. Chopping, roasting, then powdering the dried root makes an excellent coffee substitute.

ECHINACEA
Echinacea angustifolia and *E. purpurea*

Parts used: root.
Properties: antibiotic, immune tonic, blood and lymph purifier, fever reducing.

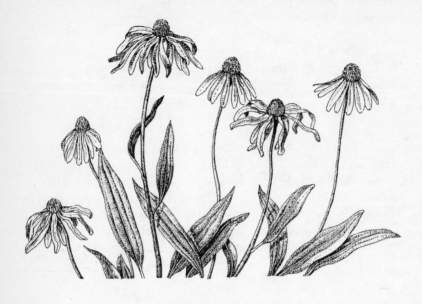

Figure 4   Echinacea

Energy: cooling, tonifying, dispersing. Reduces Fire and Water, increases Air.

Echinacea has grown in importance only relatively recently. A native of the plains region of the western United States, it was used by American Indians. The Germans have done extensive research on it in modern times and found it to be perhaps the most powerful natural antibiotic. It not only kills bacteria and viruses but actually strengthens immunity by increasing the number of white blood cells in the blood stream, thereby building immune strength. It can be used as a safe alternative to synthetic antibiotics. Echinacea is most conveniently taken in powder or tincture form, 2 capsules or 1 tsp every hour at the first sign of a cold, flu or fever or whenever antibiotic action is called for: pus, eczema, gangrene, poisonous bites (snakes, insects), poison from plants (poison ivy), infections. It can be combined with chaparral and golden seal for this purpose. It is also effective against vaginal yeast infections, candida, urinary tract and skin infections.

ELDERFLOWER
Sambucus nigra

Parts used: berries, leaves, flowers.
Properties: diaphoretic, expectorant, diuretic.
Energy: cooling, dispersing. Reduces Fire and Water, stabilizes Air.

The elder tree is another generous gift to humanity as several parts give relief in many conditions. The fragrant flowers make an excellent diaphoretic tea for use in colds, flu and fevers. Their action is enhanced by combining with peppermint or ginger and lemon. They make a delicious cordial, mixed with citrus lemon, lime or orange, which can be drunk hot in the winter or cool in summer. The ripe berries make an excellent cough syrup and the leaves can be made into an ointment for skin complaints.

FENNEL
Foeniculum vulgare

Parts used: seeds.
Properties: diuretic, demulcent, carminative.
Energy: warming, softening, moistening, balancing. Increases digestive Fire while reducing excess Fire, reduces Water, stablizes Air. Balances all three humours.
Caution: avoid prolonged or concentrated use during first trimester of pregnancy. Safe for occasional tea, culinary and short-term uses.

Fennel is an easily available culinary herb with good medicinal value. It improves digestion and thus helps clear toxic accumulations from the system. It is diuretic and helps remove excess damp and fat from the system. For gas, cramp or colitis upsets combine it with catnip, licorice, or anise. Fennel tea can be used externally to calm any skin inflammation. The seeds should be decocted, or powdered before infusing. Fennel can be used by all three constitutional types.

GARLIC
Allium sativum

Part used: corms.
Properties: circulatory stimulant, antiseptic, blood purifier, diaphoretic, digestive stimulant, carminative, expectorant, tonic.
Energy: warming, stimulating, sweet. Reduces Water and grounds excessive Air, increases digestive Fire.
Caution: avoid prolonged concentrated use during first trimester of pregnancy. Safe for occasional tea, culinary and short-term uses.

Garlic should be found in every home. Used regularly, it is an overall tonic for the system, helping to promote good digestion and assimilation, and strengthening the adrenal glands. It stimulates and improves blood circulation, because it clears cholesterol and other impurities from the blood; so it finds a place in treating excess weight, lymphatic congestion as well as hypertension and heart disease. However, it should be avoided in any bleeding conditions, such as excessive menstrual bleeding or blood in the stools. Garlic is a natural antibiotic. Eating a clove raw or expressing the juice into 1 tbs vegetable oil at the first sign of a cold, flu, or any infection will usually clear or at least weaken it. Good quality garlic powder can be used instead, though it will not be quite as effective.

GINGER
Zingiber officinalis

Part used: rhizome.
Properties: circulatory stimulant, antispasmodic, antiseptic, diaphoretic, expectorant, carminative, analgesic.
Energy: warming, slightly drying, relaxing. Reduces excess Water (mucous); stimulates digestive Fire. Clears excess Fire and calms Air.

This common culinary spice is a virtual treasure trove because it benefits such a wide variety of conditions. Its aroma instantly calms and purifies. Both powder and fresh ginger are used but bear in mind that powdered ginger is hotter and more drying than fresh. An instant massage oil can be made by grating the fresh root and mixing the juice with a little vegetable oil. This will ease the stiffness and pain of arthritis or any cramping or muscular tension. A small piece used regularly in cooking improves the digestibility of foods, especially meats, and thus helps maintain health.

By combining ginger powder with a little water and flour a paste is created for externally applying to headaches or pain anywhere. As an antispasmodic, ginger finds a place in treating intestinal or menstrual cramps and tension generally. A little ginger can be added to almost any herbal combination to ensure circulation and good penetration to tissues. It blends well with other diaphoretics to treat colds, flu and fevers. It relieves stomach upsets, belching, gas and nausea, particularly nausea during pregnancy or while travelling. It helps clear stagnant mucous congestion in the lung area. To improve its action, Water types should mix it with honey, Fire types with dark, raw sugar and Air types with salt.

GINSENG, See Special Oriental Herbs, p.139.

GOLDEN SEAL
Hydrastis canadensis

Parts used: root.
Properties: antibiotic, blood purifying, antipyretic, bitter stomach tonic, astringent, emmenagogue, laxative.
Energy: cooling and drying. Lowers high Fire, cleanses congested Water (mucous), increases Air.
Caution: This herb is not suitable for prolonged use due to a possible tendency to imbalance intestinal flora. It is best avoided during the first trimester of pregnancy because its effect on the uterus may increase the chance of a miscarriage.

This Appalachian wild flower is literally worth its weight in gold, as its name suggests. It is expensive to purchase but well worth

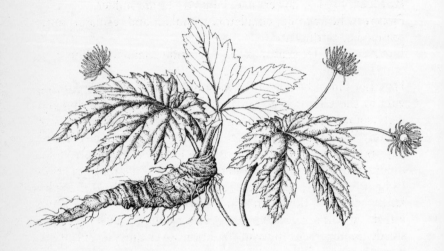

Figure 5   Golden Seal

it as it so efficiently deals with many problems; a little goes a long way. One keynote of effectiveness for golden seal is mucous membrane – that thin layer of protection which lines much of the body including the entire respiratory, digestive, urinary and reproductive tracts; others are inflammation and infection.

Golden seal deals with such ailments as colds and flu, respiratory catarrh; infections, inflammation in the stomach and intestines (ulcers, nausea, colitis, irritable bowel, gastro-enteritis); vaginal and urinary tract infections, skin eruptions, boils and infections in wounds. At the same time as healing the symptoms in these organs and tissues, golden seal actually tones them and improves their function for the future. Its bitter properties purge and strengthen the stomach, liver and bowels. Golden seal combines well with echinacea for a natural effective antibiotic.

Because of its astringent properties, golden seal should be avoided in the first three months of pregnancy as its contracting effect on the uterus may contribute to a miscarriage, if one is threatening.

HAWTHORN
Crataegus oxycantha (C. laevigata)

Part used: berries, flowers may be used but are milder.
Properties: heart tonic, circulatory stimulant and regulator, antispasmodic, astringent.
Energy: warm. Decreases excess Air while stimulating Fire.

Hawthorn must be one of the most abundant herbs still growing wild in the UK. It is certainly one of the glories of spring and early summer to see the hedgerows cascading with streams of white blossoms. In autumn the berries brighten many a dull day. Both flowers and berries used to be eaten by country folk; a conserve was made of the berries. There is a strong tradition in British herbal medicine for using hawthorn as a heart remedy. Unlike digitalis, derived from foxgloves, it is not used for acute attacks; it will not compensate for heart failure. But it does offer steady improvement in weak conditions over time; its effects are cumulative.

Hawthorn increases coronary circulation. It strengthens the heart muscle cells, nourishes them and increases energy, without overstimulating. It increases the force of the beat but not the rate. Hawthorn also evens irregular and arrhythmic heartbeat. It has antispasmodic and nervine qualities. Its most obvious use is as part of the treatment for hypertension and tachycardia. It is safe to use with the elderly who are beginning to experience loss of function. Those passing from middle to older age should consider using it on a regular, periodic basis as part of tonification and rejuvenation therapy.

HOP
Humulus lupulus

Part used: flowers.
Properties: nervine (calming, sleep inducing), bitter digestive, tonic, pain relieving.
Energy: cooling. Decreases excited Air while strengthening digestive Fire to enhance the digestion and assimilation of food energy. Coolness will aggravate Air in the long term so Air types should be sure to combine it with a warming herb for balanced effect.

Hop flowers are a well-known ingredient in both beers and herb pillows – and justifiably so. The tradition that ales and stouts will strengthen weak individuals is explained by the bitter principles in hops which act to stimulate the digestive enzymes and therefore increase nutrition. The nervine properties enhance sleep, which gives the body time to rest and repair, so hops are often found in herb pillows. Recent studies show a hormone-regulating action which improves reproductive function in both men and women. This confirms traditional lore of its effects on young girls harvesting hops. For sleeplessness, simply brew a tea before bedtime or make a herb pillow. For sleep combine hops with lime flowers, or chamomile. Externally a hop poultice or wash will cool and relieve pain and inflammation.

HORSETAIL
Equisetum arvense

Parts used: stem and leaves.
Properties: astringent, diuretic, diaphoretic, blood purifying.

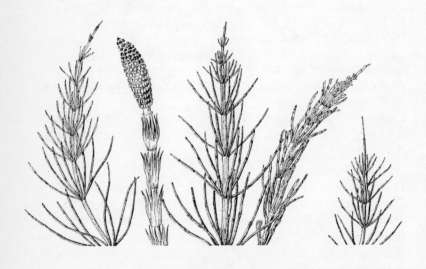

Figure 6   Horsetail

Energy: cooling, drying. Removes excess Water (damp), lowers and purges excess Fire from the blood. Increases Air so prolonged use in those tending to dryness is not recommended.

This plant really does look like a horse's tail with its bony stem and hair-like leaves. It is one of the most ancient plants, dating back to the age of dinosaurs.

Horsetail grows in damp places and traditional medicine holds that plants in such habitats are often the most effective for treating problems of fluid retention; they drain the damp collecting in the body (mushrooms are another example). Horsetail is primarily a diuretic and used for lymphatic congestion, bladder infections, cystitis, and kidney stone. It also acts to cleanse the liver and gall bladder and its diaphoretic action is useful to lower fevers as in flu or infections. Horsetail is high in silica which helps break-up calcium deposited in tissues (urinary stones, or around joints) with an equally good amount of natural calcium which nourishes bones and nerve tissue. Also known as 'scouring brush' its abrasive qualities inspired its use for scouring pots and polishing furniture.

HYSSOP
Hyssopus officinalis

Parts used: flowering stem.
Properties: aromatic, diaphoretic, anti-infectious, circulatory stimulant, expectorant, nervine.
Energy: warming, drying. Reduces excess or stagnant Water (phlegm, mucous); mildly increases Fire; calms and regulates Air.

Hyssop is a cleansing herb, especially of the respiratory tract. Traditionally associated with spiritual purity and cleanliness in the Old Testament, like all aromatic plants it is a powerful germicide and was once used to deter insects and vermin from homes and skin. Its mucous-clearing and nervine properties give it a place in treating bronchial congestion and even asthma. By releasing stagnation, it promotes the smooth flow of Vital Energy, especially that derived from Air.

JUNIPER
Juniperus communis

Parts used: berries, stem.
Properties: diuretic, carminative, diaphoretic, blood-purifying, anti-infectious, tonic.
Energy: warming, drying. Reduces excess Water, purges excess Fire and stimulates digestive Fire; warming to Air types at the same time it clears excess Air humour.
Caution: Do not use in cases of nephritis (chronic kidney inflammation). Avoid prolonged concentrated use during first trimester of pregnancy.

Juniper berries are a common culinary flavouring. They improve the digestibility of such foods as cabbage. They are also used in the distillation of gin.

Juniper's primary areas of action are on the digestive and urinary systems. Its warm, aromatic qualities aid digestion. It both stimulates the diuretic action of the kidneys and warms the circulation, helping to eliminate excess damp and cold. It also strengthens the adrenal glands. It finds a place in treating water retention, lymphatic congestion, arthritis, gout, rheumatism, stones, cystitis and bladder infections. However if the kidneys are highly inflamed as in nephritis, do not use it; its warming qualities may aggravate the heat in inflammations.

KELP
Fucus vesiculosis

Parts used: leaves.
Properties: tonic, nourishing, demulcent, expectorant, diuretic. High in minerals and vitamins; a natural supplement.
Energy: cooling and moistening. Tonifies bodily fluids.
Caution: avoid self-medication in conditions of hyperthyroidism, heart and kidney disease, lung abcesses and TB.

Kelp and other seaweeds are the great gifts from the sea. Kelp carries all the positive qualities of the sea, strengthening the fluid base of the body, the water from which life springs and in which it thrives. The iodine in kelp nourishes the thyroid gland and so maintains good metabolism and glandular function. Its moistening qualities help it to dissolve and remove stagnations such as tumours and cysts, and catarrh in the respiratory tract in the form of sore throat or cough. While strengthening the fluids, kelp's diuretic action helps drain water or excess damp. It well illustrates the regulating and balancing effect herbs have on the body in general. Take kelp tablets as a daily supplement and when you want to use it medicinally just grind them to a powder to blend with other herbs.

LEMON BALM
Melissa officinalis

Part used: leaves, flowering stem.
Properties: diaphoretic, stimulant, carminative, antiseptic, circulates energy. Blood purifier, uterine tonic and blood regulator.
Energy: cooling and balancing. Calms Air, reduces Fire, clears stagnant Water, and clarifies the mind.

This herb's name says it all: the uplifting, purifying zest of lemon and a balm to troubles, whether those of a depressed mind, an upset stomach or an insect-bitten skin. Its Latin name, *Melissa* – from the Greek for honey – tells us it is loved by bees, who always seem to know the best healing plants in any vicinity. A women's friend, it can be used to ease cramps and pre-menstrual congestion and depression.

LICORICE
Glycyrrhiza glabra

Parts used: root.
Properties: demulcent, expectorant, digestive, mild laxative, tonic, nourishing, harmonizing.
Energy: neutral, moistening. Harmonizing. Strengthens vital

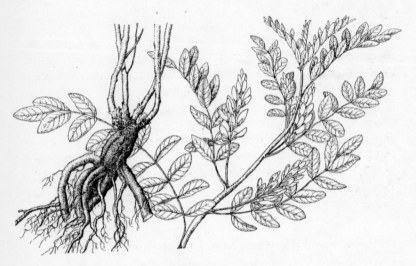

Figure 7   Licorice

body fluids (Water). Reduces excess damp and phlegm. Strengthens digestive Fire while lowering inflammation, calms Air.
Caution: avoid in conditions of water retention, oedema, cardiovascular disease.

Known in Chinese medicine as the Peacemaker, licorice holds a special place in herbal medicine; it has a smoothing, soothing effect and delicious flavour. It can be added to blends to harmonize the energies of the other herbs and buffer their effects. With its sweet, nutritive qualities it benefits weakness and hypoglycaemia. It promotes hormone balance and benefits women at times such as puberty, pregnancy and menopause. Its demulcent, expectorant properties and appealing taste give it a prime place in treating coughs and congestion in the respiratory tract, especially in children. It can be made into a cough syrup, or used as a decoction. Coming from the rhizome of the plant, licorice imparts an earthy grounding quality when the Air humour is upset or imbalanced, for example in cramps or spasm. However it should not be used by those suffering from hypertension with fluid retention or oedema.

MARIGOLD
Calendula officinalis

Parts used: flowers.
Properties: anti-inflammatory, blood purifying, diaphoretic, astringent, healing.
Energy: cooling, soothing. Counters excess Fire, as in inflammation, and calms irritated Air (itching).

Marigolds are among the most charming of flowers and should be in every garden; they quickly seed themselves and will grace your home year after year. Visually their very shape and colour capture and reflect the optimism and brightness of the sun and summer.

Marigold is used to quell excess fire in the form of inflammation. It soothes skin abrasions, burns, stings and bites. Have a pot of calendula ointment on hand in the first aid kit to soothe and promote the mending of tissue. Marigold tea is used for circulating energy and blood to dispel bruising, to regulate menses, as a diaphoretic to clear the heat of fevers and eruptive skin complaints. It combines well with comfrey or chickweed in oils or ointments.

MARSHMALLOW
Malva species

Parts used: root, leaves.
Properties: demulcent, anti-inflammatory, mucilage, blood purifying, astringent.
Energy: cooling and moistening. Increases Water, reduces Fire and Air. Strengthens vital fluids and lubricates tissue.

Just touching the leaves and flowers of marshmallow gives a clue to its qualities; they are soft and slightly thicker than most. Marshmallow, like slippery elm and comfrey, contains an abundance of mucilage which, when combined with water, swells to form a soft spongy mass. When any tissue in the body is inflamed or irritated, reach for marshmallow root. It is used for the pain and irritation of kidney stones combined with diuretics, irritable bowel or colitis combined with laxatives, for the bronchial passages combined with expectorants.

Marshmallow root is nourishing and can be used as a nutritional supplement in weakness and convalescence. Hollyhocks and other wild mallows have similar but milder properties.

MEADOWSWEET
Filipendula ulmaria

Parts used: flowers and leaves.
Properties: nervine (analgesic, antispasmodic), astringent, diaphoretic, diuretic.
Energy: cooling, drying. Reduces excess Water, calms aggravated Air, cools Fire.

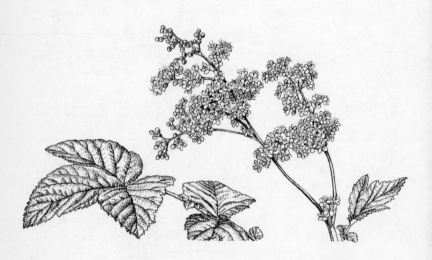

Figure 8   Meadowsweet

This beautiful wayside herb with its clusters of soft, creamy and sweet smelling flowers and red-based stems, is a good source of natural aspirin. It contains salicylic compounds, from which aspirin was originally synthesized. It can be used as a natural anti-inflammatory and analgesic for headaches and acid stomach, for arthritic and rheumatic pains and urinary infections. Its other properties help dry excess damp in the system which often lies behind these conditions. White willow bark can be used similarly.

MINTS
Mentha species

Parts used: leaves, flowering stem.
Properties: carminative, stimulating, circulates energy, diaphoretic, liver cleansing, mucous reducing.
Energy: warming and cooling, drying with prolonged use. Balancing. Reduces Water, cools excess Fire but promotes digestion. Calms Air.
Caution: avoid prolonged concentrated use during first trimester of pregnancy. Safe for occasional tea, culinary and short-term uses.

The mints form a large group within the *Labatiae* family and the majority of them are excellent medicinals. Their stimulating quality is unusual in being both energizing and calming at the same time. Their action is gentle yet still very effective for the stomach, liver, nerves, blood and lymph circulation. They grow easily in gardens or on windowsills and should find a place in every home.

Peppermint (*Mentha piperita*) is the most strongly stimulating of the mints. It is actually a hybrid between pennyroyal (*M. pulegium*) and spearmint (*M. spicata*) and is sterile. It is excellent combined with elderflower for the first sign of cold or flu, or fever. As a digestive aid it helps sooth the stomach-based form of headache. Many find it an acceptable substitute for coffee, giving that extra pick-up without the harmful side effects. Its initial pungency stimulates metabolism and is followed by a mild coolness which refreshes, making its overall action balancing to all three humours. Excessive use however, may eventually dry and aggravate Air. Spearmint is very similar to peppermint, though milder, and horsemint (M. *arvensis*) is also used.

MULLEIN
Verbascum thapsus

Parts used: leaves, flowers.
Properties: demulcent, astringent, diuretic, nervine.
Energy: cooling and drying. Reduces excess Water, calms and nourishes excited Air, cools Fire.

Mullein is a visually striking plant with its tall stem rising straight and breaking out into yellow blooms at the end. The leaves too are unusual: soft, broad and fuzzy, roseate in form, they remind one of a comfortable woolly blanket. Mulleins are often seen standing along highways like sentinels.

Mullein is primarily used for treating inflammations and swellings, especially when lymph nodes in the throat, neck,

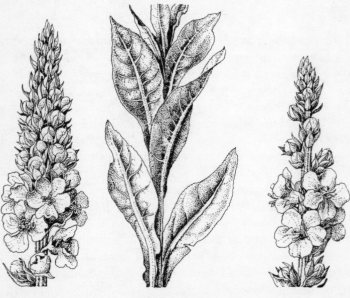

Figure 9   Mullein

arms and groin swell or are congested as in sore throats, mumps and fluid in the ear. It cleanses the lymphatic system generally. For this it is applied as a poultice and taken as a tea. Its mucous reducing properties make it useful for coughs and catarrh. It also has nervine-anodyne properties which relieve pain and promote sound sleep. Mullein tea will arrest diarrhoea.

For ear ache, make a herbal oil with mullein, soak a piece of cotton wool in it and place it in the ear. For Air types or for excited Air humour, infuse mullein with hot milk and drink at night before sleeping.

NETTLE
Urtica urens

Parts used: leaves and stem.
Properties: blood purifying, circulatory stimulant, nourishing, tonic, astringent, blood regulating (haemostatic).
Energy: cooling. Cools excess Fire while strengthening circulation. Reduces excess Water. Calms and nourishes Air.

This prickly herb which bedevils the walker in the wild and in some gardens is the botanical equivalent of a treasure guarded by a dragon. Beyond those stinging hairs nettle is a blood cleanser and circulatory stimulant, rich in iron and other minerals. The tender young leaves may be steamed like spinach as a pot-herb. It finds a place in regulating and strengthening the blood generally, for anaemia and bleeding. It clears excess damp and so helps with arthritis and rheumatism, and with asthma and lung congestion. Its astringency and haemostatic properties signal it for diarrhoea, dysentery and excess menstrual flow. Taken regularly as a tonic tea, it helps maintain health.

OREGON GRAPE
Mahonia aquifolium

Parts used: root.
Properties: blood purifying, tonifying (liver), laxative, antiseptic.
Energy: cooling. Reduces excess Fire, reduces excess Water, regulates and stabilizes Air.

Caution: Avoid prolonged concentrated use during first trimester of pregnancy. Safe for occasional tea, culinary and short-term uses.

Many gardens in Britain display this North American import, known as the holly-leaved barberry, without their owners appreciating its outstanding qualities as a liver cleanser and tonifier, blood purifier, laxative and bowel cleanser. Its Eurasian cousin, the common barberry (*Berberis vulgaris*), a shrub found in hedgerows and waysides, is used similarly, though its action is milder. The berries were once commonly eaten and prepared as condiments.

The bitter taste stimulates gastric juices, improving the digestion and assimilation of food, and purges the liver. Oregon grape and barberry are used for cases of hepatitis, jaundice, constipation, diabetes and arthritis. Another use is in problems due to congestion of vital energy, such as moodiness or irritability as for example in pre-menstrual tension or depression. It may be combined with turmeric for this purpose.

PARSLEY
Petroselinum crispum

Parts used: leaves, root.
Properties: diuretic, tonic, carminative, nutritive, emmenagogue.
Energy: warming, stimulating. Reduces excess Water, and calms Air. Aggravates excess Fire when used in excess.
Caution: Avoid prolonged concentrated use during first trimester of pregnancy. Safe for occasional tea, culinary and short-term uses.

Most people don't realize how healing parsley is. The root is stronger than the leaves and better for more severe conditions. Parsley improves digestion and assimilation of food. It is an excellent diuretic and will help the body expel stones. It eases menstrual cramp, headache and tension. It supplies valuable minerals and vitamins and can be used regularly as a health tonic. However, in cases of inflammation of the kidneys it should not be used unless combined with marshmallow root.

PLANTAIN
Plantago major

Parts used: leaves.
Properties: diuretic, blood purifying, astringent, demulcent.
Energy: cooling. Reduces excess Fire and Water, relieves congested Air.

Plantain is one of the most common European weeds, often aggressively driven out of lawns. Native American Indians noticed that wherever Europeans had lived this new plant appeared and named it white-man's foot. They were also quick to appreciate its properties and used it to counter the poisons of snakebite. Do allow some to remain in a corner of your garden so you may have instant access for relief of insect stings, skin infections, wounds, abrasions, and burns. For a first aid poultice, simply chew the leaf for a moment and apply to the skin; for longer term treatment wash the area daily with plantain tea.

Used internally in tea form, plantain clears toxins from the blood which give rise to urinary infections, hepatitis and feverish conditions as well as chronic skin complaints such as eczema. Another common weed, cleavers, is similarly diuretic. The seeds of *Plantago indica*, psyllium seeds, are commonly used as a bulk laxative.

RASPBERRY
Rubus idaeus

Parts used: leaves.
Properties: astringent, tonic (uterus and stomach), blood regulating (haemostatic and menstrual regulator), mild blood purifier.
Energy: cooling, cleansing. Reduces excess Fire and Water, calms Air but can aggravate if used excessively.

The native European wild raspberry has rightly been woman's best friend and used to strengthen the uterus for pregnancy and childbirth. But its use need not stop once the baby has arrived. Its stomachic properties also help allay nausea and it cleans the stomach and intestines. It should be more generally used by everyone. It is high in vitamin C, manganese, iron and other nutrients and can be used regularly as a general tonic. Its mild but effective astringent and blood purifying actions also clear excess mucous and heat toxins, so use it for colds, flu, sore throats as well as diarrhoea and dysentery, especially in children. Raspberry is often the most easily available and effective treatment for menstrual cramp, heavy or irregular periods and vaginal discharge. Combine it with a little ginger to enhance both flavour and action.

Related herbs with similar properties are wild strawberry and blackberry.

RED CLOVER
Trifolium pratense

Parts used: flowers.
Properties: blood purifying, tonic, nutritive, expectorant, antibiotic.
Energy: cooling, tonifying. Clears excess Fire, reduces excess Water.

A small, humble and beautiful wildflower, red clover is the glory of summer meadows and one of the most useful and effective herbal medicines. It is a major ingredient in a famous cancer formula for it cleanses the blood (and thus tissues generally) and is deeply nourishing to the body with its abundance of minerals. It can be taken as a tea for respiratory complaints and mild fevers especially when the person is young, elderly or debilitated. Use the tea externally for any troublesome skin problem that refuses to heal. For antibiotic action, combine it with others such as chaparral or echinacea.

ROSEMARY
Rosmarinus officinalis

Parts used: leaves.
Properties: aromatic-antiseptic, carminative, nervine-analgesic, circulatory stimulant, diaphoretic, blood regulator (emmenagogue).
Energy: warming, dispersing. Clears excess Fire, reduces excess Water, relieves irritated Air.

Caution: avoid prolonged concentrated use during first trimester of pregnancy. Safe for occasional tea, culinary and short-term uses.

Reach for rosemary as a convenient treatment for many common complaints. Use it for stomach aches, headaches, symptoms of flu, cold or fever and congestion such as constipation or pre-menstrual build-up. Use it generously in cooking to keep the system clean and free.

SAGE
Salvia officinalis

Parts used: leaves.
Properties: astringent, aromatic-antiseptic, stimulant, diuretic, carminative, expectorant.
Energy: warming, dispersing, drying. Clears excess Water and Fire, but may aggravate excess Air (nervousness, dryness).
Caution: avoid prolonged concentrated use during first trimester of pregnancy. Safe for occasional tea, culinary and short-term uses. *Contraindications*: nursing mothers.

Sage has very strong astringent and drying properties which indicate its use to clear excess mucous from the nose and lungs, drain sores and ulcers and control bleeding. It is most specifically effective for swollen, sore throats used as a tea and gargle. Another indication is to allay hot flushes during the menopause; for this it can be mixed with rosemary, skullcap and raspberry leaves or motherwort.

The same actions mean sage should be avoided by nursing mothers, unless of course it is necessary to stop nursing. For this purpose, drink the tea and apply as a fomentation.

SASSAFRAS
Sassafras albidum

Parts used: bark of the root.
Properties: blood purifying, diaphoretic, diuretic, tonic (liver), astringent, stimulant.
Energy: warming.

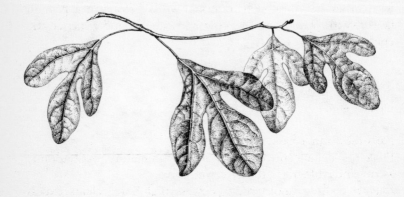

Figure 10   Sassafras

Caution: avoid in strong, acute inflammatory conditions and for long-term use.

The sassafras tree grows abundantly throughout the south-eastern United States and is much used by Native American and country folk there. The bark is deliciously aromatic and flavours the famous root beer beloved by southerners. A spring tonic tea was traditionally brewed to cleanse the blood and system generally.

Sassafras is most commonly used to treat arthritis, rheumatism and skin complaints as well as colds and flu, where its blood purifying and damp-removing actions give the benefit.

SKULLCAP
Scutellaria lateriflora

Parts used: flowering stem, leaves.
Properties: nervine. Antispasmodic, relaxing, sedative; anti-inflammatory.
Energy: cooling. Reduces excess Fire; calms and regulates Air.

Skullcap is a reliable, safe nervine for promoting sound sleep and relaxing and restoring the body during stress. It is helpful during drug detoxification to counter the discomforts and anxieties of withdrawal. High in minerals which nourish the nervous tissue, skullcap can be used safely for hypertension, convulsions, epilepsy and neuralgia. It is usually combined with other nervines such as hops, wood betony and passion flower, with perhaps a little ginger to balance and enhance the energy.

SLIPPERY ELM
Ulmus rubra

Parts used: inner bark.
Properties: demulcent, nutritive, anti-inflammatory, expectorant, astringent, vulnerary, tonic, carminative.
Energy: cooling, moistening. Lowers high Fire, clears excess Water (mucous) while strengthening vital fluid base, stabilizes Air.

Slippery elm is one of the most useful herbs and should always be kept on hand. It benefits conditions ranging from superficial wounds and ulcerations to medium level respiratory congestion, constipation, diarrhoea, and colitis, to chronic wasting diseases where there is dryness and weakness.

Slippery elm has an abundance of mucilage which, when mixed with water, thickens and holds the moisture. Whenever tissues are inflamed and irritated, such as in sore throat, stomach acidity or ulcers, bronchitis and asthma, irritable bowel, colitis or gastro-enteritis, picture this herb spreading its thick, soothing and softening coat over them. For sore throat, take it as a tea and gargle to ensure contact with the tissues. For stomach and gastro-intestinal problems also take as tea, perhaps mixed with a little cinnamon or cloves for flavour and enhanced effect. Use a little in poultices, even if it is not specifically indicated, for it makes the perfect base to hold the other herbs. Carry some when travelling for use on minor wounds, stings and abrasions or tummy bugs, and for both diarrhoea and constipation.

The tawny-coloured, somewhat fibrous powder is made into

a gruel to sustain and strengthen those debilitated with age or chronic, exhausting illnesses and even infants that are not thriving. It builds health and the vital base fluids which sustain the body. Marshmallow root is used very similarly, though it has a special affinity for problems of the urinary tract.

ST JOHN'S WORT
Hypericum perforatum

Parts used: leaves, flowers.
Properties: blood purifying, anti-inflammatory, nervine: sedative, anti-depressant, tonic and pain relieving; wound healing.
Energy: cooling, calming. Decreases excess Fire and Air.

Named for the fact that it blooms around the summer solstice – St John's tide – this once common European wildflower has a long history of use in herbal medicine but recently new applications have been discovered. It was traditionally used to treat wounds, inflammations and ulcers, both internal and external, and painful sciatica, neuralgia and rheumatism. For this latter purpose the beautiful red massage oil is produced by macerating the flowers in vegetable oil for six weeks. (The flowers are yellow but contain a red pigment which shows in the oil.) This can also be taken internally a tablespoonful at a time.

More recently it has been found to be an effective anti-depressant, lifting and lightening the mood; also effective for anxiety, including night terror in children. It can be used to treat such symptoms in menopause. Another contemporary application which is showing results is in the treatment of AIDS; it is prescribed for its nervine and anti-viral (blood purifying) effects.

THYME
Thymus vulgaris

Part used: leaves, flowers.
Properties: diaphoretic, nervine, stimulant, carminative, respiratory and lymph cleanser, antiseptic.
Energy: warming, calming. Reduces excess Water, calms Air, clears Fire.

Caution: Avoid prolonged concentrated use during first trimester of pregnancy. Safe for occasional tea, culinary and short-term uses.

There are many varieties of thyme but common thyme (*Thymus vulgaris*) is best medicinally. Thyme is excellent when put to work at the first signs of colds or flu, and for any respiratory complaints, coughs and sore throats. It stimulates metabolism and strengthens nerves.

TURMERIC
Curcuma longa

Parts used: rhizome.
Properties: blood purifying and liver tonic, antibacterial, astringent, carminative, vulnerary.
Energy: warming. Reduces excess Fire while strengthening digestion; clears excess Water.

This very common Indian aromatic of striking yellow colour is in fact a medicine with remarkable powers, so keep your kitchen supply of good quality. Turmeric kills bacteria, counteracts toxins in the blood, cleanses and improves liver function. Apply turmeric paste or a poultice externally to wounds, stings, and skin infections or boils, mixed with a little slippery elm. Take it internally as part of a blood purifying blend, with red clover, chaparral, and/or echinacea for skin problems such as acne.

In India it is used not only in curry blends but also to treat even severe blood toxicity and stagnation such as gangrene. Current research shows it has anti-tumour properties. Turmeric can be used regularly in cooking as a purifying carminative which will aid complete digestion and assimilation, and maintain good health as well as making dishes visually attractive.

VALERIAN
Valeriana officinalis

Part used: root.
Properties: nervine: sedative, relaxant, antispasmodic, analgesic, tonic; diuretic.

Energy: cooling. Calms and stabilizes disturbed Air, while nourishing nerve tissue. Mildly reduces excess Water.

Valerian is a native European herb which has seen centuries of use. It should not be confused with the red valerian (*Centranthus ruber*). The strong aroma – isovaleric acid is the main active constituent – in the roots develops on drying so it is best used when dried. Valerian roots are high in calcium, which nourishes the nerve tissue and helps it recover from stress. Many people do not like the fragrance of valerian, but it is attractive to cats and other mammals, and cats will instinctively eat the plant when injured; it helps recovery from shock, is antibacterial and healing.

Valerian is a major herb for the nervous system. It helps the body cope and recover from stress. It relaxes and induces sound sleep. Traditional uses include treatment for hysteria, vertigo, fainting and irritability. Its antispasmodic action helps with muscle and menstrual cramps. Valerian benefits athletes and anyone engaged in aerobics and weight training, as part

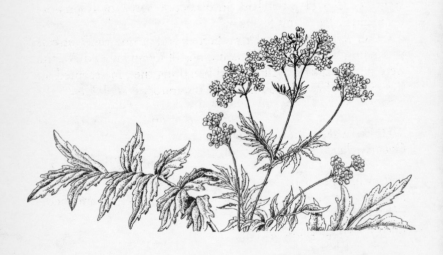

Figure 11   *Valerian*

of preventative and recovery treatment. The powder may be combined with a little ginger, lemon balm or hops and taken as a tea to treat insomnia, cramps and stress.

A relative of valerian, spikenard, has been used since classical times in the Middle East, being part of the oil used for anointing in the Old Testament. It is also used medicinally in India.

WHITE PINE BARK
Pinus albicaulis (strobus)

Parts used: inner bark, young needles.
Properties: aromatic, antibacterial, stimulating, expectorant, blood purifying, diaphoretic.
Energy: warming, stimulating. Clears excess Fire, reduces excess Water.

The white pine of North America is one of the most beautiful trees. It was much used by native American Indians for both food and medicine, the new pine tops having been eaten as a spring tonic, the resin tea used for sore throats and as an expectorant. White pine bark is a major ingredient in the famous Composition Powder developed by Thomsonian herbalism to energize the body and overcome fevers, infections and stagnation. Use the young needles or inner bark in decoction form for respiratory complaints, colds and fevers.

Other pines have similar properties and at one time retreats to sanatoriums in the pine mountains of Germany and Austria were justly popular; walking and breathing the pine-scented air was curative for asthma and other respiratory complaints.

WHITE OAK
Quercus alba

Part used: inner bark.
Properties: astringent, blood regulating, haemostatic, antibacterial, vulnerary.
Energy: drying, cooling.

The bark of the white and other oaks is high in calcium and tannins which make it useful for any condition of flaccidity and flux, such as diarrhoea, worms, leucorrhoea, bleeding. It tightens and strengthens any tissue, especially bone, and promotes healing of wounds. Acorns – gathered, roasted and ground – make an excellent coffee substitute. Walnut leaves have like properties.

WHITE WILLOW
Salix alba

Part used: inner bark.
Properties: nervine – analgesic pain reliever; blood purifying – anti-inflammatory, antibacterial; astringent.
Energy: cooling. Clears excess Fire, soothes and stabilizes Air, reduces Water.

White willow bark has traditionally been the natural aspirin, used by native American Indians and white settlers to treat acute pain and inflammation of fevers and arthritis. It treats the symptoms while clearing the underlying causes of congestion and stagnation. Take it powdered in capsules, tablets or brewed as tea. European willows have similar properties.

WILD YAM
Dioscorea villosa and *D. batata*

Part used: root.
Properties: tonic – liver and reproductive tissue; nervine – antispasmodic; diaphoretic, diuretic, expectorant.
Energy: warming. Reduces excess Fire and Water; calms irritated Air; strengthens vital fluids.

The Mexican and Central American wild yam provides the source material from which the birth-control pill, cortisones and sex hormones are derived. Yams are high in plant hormones which can be synthesized by the body to support its own hormone health. Thus, wild yam root is an important constituent of hormone-regulating, herbal formulas. In addition it is antispasmodic, diuretic and liver cleansing. It can be used to relieve skin problems like eczema as well as muscular and menstrual cramps and the symptoms of congestion which precede the period. It is a sweet, nutritive tonic food treatment for weakness and wasting.

Yam is also good for digestive problems as it relieves wind and stagnation of the liver and gall bladder. As an antispasmodic, it can also be used for neuralgic pain.

YARROW
Achillea millefolium

Part used: leaves and flowers.
Properties: aromatic, bactericidal, diaphoretic, anti-inflammatory, astringent; blood regulating (haemostatic, tonic and emmenagogue).
Energy: warming, drying. Clears excess Fire and Water from blood and digestive tract.

Yarrow has been used continuously since well before the Christian era. Its Latin name is from Achilles, the hero who could only

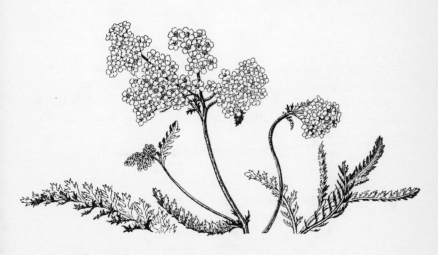

Figure 12   Yarrow

be wounded in his heel, and the ancient Greeks used yarrow as a wound healing herb. Like plantain, it was taken to the Americas on the feet of settlers and the Indians soon appreciated its uses and found new ones as a blood tonic and regulator given to women after childbirth.

Yarrow clears excess damp mucous from the digestive tract and its diaphoretic and anti-inflammatory action makes it ideal for expelling colds and flu before they take hold. Like all herbs rich in aromatic essential oils, it kills infections and may be used as a tea or poultice on wounds and bleeding. Women may take it as a blood regulating tonic to ease cramps and excessive bleeding. It especially benefits Fire and Water types and may be combined with peppermint for colds, with chamomile for digestive and nerve-calming purposes.

SPECIAL ORIENTAL HERBS

The following herbs are among several outstanding herbs that have been in use in Chinese or Indian medicine for thousands of years and have recently become more well known in the West. Their value is confirmed by scientific research.

DONG QUAI (or DANG GUI)
Angelica sinensis

Part used: root.
Properties: blood regulating, emmenagogue and tonic, antispasmodic, diaphoretic.
Energy: warming, tonifying. Clears excess Fire and stagnant Water, calms and regulates Air. Tonifies blood and the circulatory system.
Caution: avoid in pregnancy and with diarrhoea.

The Chinese angelica is related to our European angelica and has comparable antispasmodic properties but with important additions. As well as relaxing cramps and tension, its warming properties also clear congestion and improve circulation and its nutritive tonifying properties actually improve the quality of the blood. This makes it invaluable for women as it both eases symptoms of the monthly cycle and rebuilds the blood in its aftermath. However, it is not only for women. Dong quai benefits anyone who needs to strengthen the quality and circulation of blood – those with anaemia or symptoms of tiredness – or suffer from cramping pains and tension. It is good added to wound blends as it eases pain while improving circulation of blood to speedily resolve bruising and swelling: this makes it a good recovery medicine for any injury or surgery.

GINSENG
Panax ginseng

Parts used: root.
Properties: tonic to vital energy and immune system, adaptogen, circulatory stimulant.
Energy: warming, nutritive tonic. Revitalizes collapsed energy, combats stress. Strengthens Fire, Air and Vital fluids.
Caution: Avoid in conditions of extreme nervous anxiety, hypertension, cardiovascular disease. Those who are in robust health should restrict use to short terms. Other tonics such as *Eleuthro coccus*, *codonopsis* and tienchi (*Panax pseudoginseng*) are more appropriate for longer term tonification.

Ginseng has greatly extended the horizons of western herbalism; it seems to have reappeared at the right moment. Just as we were beginning to appreciate and understand the nature of stress and immunity, we were also (though not for the first time) opening ourselves to medicinal contributions from other cultures and especially those of China. For two thousand years or more the Chinese have appreciated the unique properties of ginseng to enable the body to deal with and recover from stress and for many other ailments. It is the single herb which, more than any other, demonstrates the concept of a Vital Energy tonic. Scientific research has confirmed its remarkable properties and prompted the coining of a new phrase 'adaptogen' to account for these. It treats fatigue, convalescence, debility, injury and shock, stress and weakened immunity, and chronic diseases.

We in the West would do well to make it a regular part of our health maintenance programme, as the Chinese do. Small amounts are added to remedies for specific organ weaknesses to enhance the effects of the overall formula and strengthen the organs, especially lungs and heart. It finds a place in treatment of AIDS and HIV.

American ginseng (*Panay quinquifolius*) also has tonic properties which are much appreciated by Chinese medicine.

ASHWAGHANDA
Withania somnifera

Parts used: root.
Properties: rejuvenative and energy tonic; nervine – sedative and tonic; astringent, vulnerary.
Energy: warming, nutritive. Calms and strengthens Air. Increases Fire. Reduces excess Water.

Ashwaghanda, which means 'that which gives the vitality of the horse', is an important tonic herb in Ayurvedic medicine and is now becoming available in the West. In Ayurveda, the concept of rejuvenating is comparable to that of energy tonic as discussed under ginseng. Ashwaghanda is similar to ginseng in that it strengthens both tissues and vital energy, especially those of the nervous system, so it is good for the treatment of wasting and deficiency (even in children); the negative effects of overwork and ageing; and for strengthening the immune system through its influence on vital and reproductive fluids. It can be taken with warm milk to promote sound sleep. It could be used as a regular health-maintaining tonic as well as added to formulas for specific weaknesses.

GOTU KOLA
Centella asiatica

Parts used: leaves and stem.
Properties: rejuvenative tonic, nervine, blood purifying, diuretic.
Energies: Clears excess Fire, reduces excess Water, strengthens and calms Air. Tonifies immunity and energy.

Gotu kola has similar properties to ashwaghanda, though it works more on the nerve, blood and marrow tissues than hormonal and reproductive fluids. It cleanses the blood, so is good for fevers and skin complaints, and calms and strengthens the nerves.

Ayurveda has a unique classification for herbs called 'satvic'. These herbs clear and calm the mind and spirit and promote the qualities needed for spiritual practice. Such herbs, including ashwaghanda, sandalwood, and gotu kola, have several properties acting at the physical level, but in addition have an extra sphere of influence, the mental and spiritual. The Indian name for gotu kola is *Brahmi*, or that which leads to knowledge of Brahman, or supreme reality. Such herbs are taken to promote tranquillity and prepare for meditation. David Frawley states that gotu kola wakens the crown *chakra*, vitalizes brain cells and balances the right and left hemispheres of the brain. For meditation, take gotu kola infusion with honey.

8

Taking it Further

I HOPE THIS BOOK has served to introduce you to the fascinating and beneficial practice of herbal medicine, and inspires you to grow and use herbs, and to protect their continued existence in the wild.

Today is an exciting time to be involved in herbal healing, not least because of the possibility for herbalism to become securely established as a primary health care service in both developed and developing nations. May all who value herbal healing contribute whatever and however they can to supporting our freedom to use herbs medicinally and for professional herbalists to practise.

TRAINING IN HERBAL MEDICINE

For readers who would like to study herbal medicine more deeply and under the guidance of a tutor there are two avenues to consider and the choice depends on your aims.

Introductory Courses

Those who want to know more in order to practise safely and successfully on themselves and their families, and to enjoy herbal medicine as an integral part of their lives by growing, processing and using their own home remedies could choose an introductory course taught by a local herbalist, perhaps under the auspices of the adult education department of their local college or secondary school. If on enquiry you find your local school does not yet offer such a course, then you could urge them to do so and drum up support for it among your friends and aquaintances.

Alternatively, you might ask a local herbalist if you could help out in some way, in the capacity of an apprentice: learning by doing, under a watchful eye.

If there is no trained herbalist in the area an alternative is to enrol in an introductory correspondence or distance-learning course offered by one of the professional teaching bodies. Almost all offer such courses and the reader may write for details to the schools.

These courses usually consist of lesson notes, suggested reading, and questions to answer along with practical assignments and the opportunity to attend three to six day seminars given by qualified tutors.

Professional Training Courses

The second avenue is for those who wish to practise herbal medicine professionally. The professional herbalist sees patients on an individual basis for their health problems and prescribes and provides herbal medicines after taking a thorough case history and conducting a diagnosis for each patient. Follow up consultations will monitor progress and allow for adjustments to the prescription. (The authority to prescribe may be limited in some countries.)

Practising as a herbalist also involves work as a herbal pharmacist, mixing and blending herbs in various preparations; as well as being a self-employed business person, with all the practicalities that involves; and continuing the study necessary to keep up to date with new developments and research in the field.

It is important to point out that at the moment the status of the professional herbalist is undergoing some challenges to its autonomy and even existence. As alternative therapies in general have become more popular and directly chosen by many more people – no longer by just a few eccentrics or those on the 'fringe'– they have begun to be noticed not only by government regulators in the interests of public safety, but also by medical physicians and pharmaceutical companies who to some extent may feel threatened by competition from herbalists and herbal medicines and may wish to undermine them.

The place of herbal medicine within the European Community

is also in the process of being clarified and defined, necessitating cooperation and compromise among the different legal statuses and practices of herbalists.

In the UK herbalists' associations are in the process of meeting together and with sympathetic MPs and MEPs in order to increase their capacity to meet these challenges and secure an established place for herbal medicine as an autonomous profession. The training institutions are evolving their training accordingly too, for example courses are being improved and some modules may be offered in conjunction with a university, thereby securing a wider academic recognition. In the US similar moves are taking place, though necessarily state by state. Similar challenges are being met and responded to in Australia and New Zealand.

At the professional level, most courses require a commitment of from three to four years of training. This may be arranged either on a part-time basis with distance learning or as full-time study. Requirements for entry may vary and an interview will be helpful in determining suitability. It is not always necessary to have higher level qualifications and people enter the profession from many different age groups.

Basic training would include study of botany and plant identification; human anatomy and physiology; pathology (disease processes) from both a Western/orthodox and a holistic/complementary perspective; herbal pharmacy and pharmacognosy (how herbs work in the body); the different herbal therapies and formulas; clinical diagnosis and consultation procedures; clinical practice under supervision; and professional ethics.

Some courses may tend to specialize in one particular tradition, for example Chinese, Western-naturopathic, or Ayurvedic (Indian).

Training Institutions

The following list details the addresses of some established training institutions. Contact these for referral to your local herbalist.

In the UK

. East-West College of Herbalism UK, Hartswood, Marsh Green, Hartfield, E. Sussex TN7 4ET. Tel 0342 282 2312.
Training in Michael Tierra's Chinese-based but eclectic approach to herbalism.

Mohsin Institute, Centre for Tibb, 446 East Park Road, Leicester LE5 5HH. Tel 0533 734633.
Training in Islamic Tibb traditional medicine.

The College of Herbs and Natural Medicine, 25 Curzon Street, Basford, Newcastle-under-Lyme, Staffordshire ST5 OPD. Tel 0782 717383.
Training based on Dr Chrisopher's approach to herbalism.

The School of Phytotherapy, Bucksteep Manor, Boodle Street Green, Hailsham, Kent BN27 4RT. Tel 0323 833812.

The Scottish School of Herbal Medicine, PO Box 52, Glasgow G4 0DT.
Introductory courses in herbal medicine at present, with profes-sional course in preparation.

Ayurvedic Network, PO Box 188, Exeter, Devon.
Publishes a newsletter and contact list, and sponsors annual seminars by Dr Vasant Lad in the UK.

In the USA

American Institute of Vedic Studies, PO Box 8357, Santa Fe, New Mexico, 87504.
Training in Ayurvedic healing.

The Ayurvedic Institute, PO Box 23445, Albuquerque, NM 87192.
Training in Ayurvedic healing.

East-West School of Herbal Studies, P.O. Box 712-H, Santa Cruz, CA 95061.
Training in Michael Tierra's approach to herbalism.

The School of Natural Medicine, PO Box 7369, Boulder, Colorado. Training in Farida Sharan's approach to herbalism.

The School of Natural Healing, Provo, Utah.
Training in Dr Christopher's approach.

The School of Herbal Medicine, PO Box 168-C, Suquamish, WA 98392.

Blazing Star Herbal School, PO Box 6HC, Shelburne Falls, MA 01370.

California School of Herbal Studies, Box 39, Forestville, CA 95439.

In Australia

Dunn's Herbal Clinic and School, 345 Badgerup Rd, Wannesco, Western Australia.

College of Herbal Medicine, Founder, Dorothy Hall, Sydney, New South Wales.

School of Phytotherapy, Registrar Pat Bone, c/o Medi-Herb, PTY Ltd, 124 MacEvoy St, Warwick, Queensland 4370.

FURTHER READING

For those who prefer to study herbal medicine at home and without the guidance of a course or a tutor, there are many excellent books and periodicals on the subject, some of which are suggested in the following list.

Christopher, Dr John, *The School of Natural Healing*, Biworld Publishing, Provo, Utah, 1976.

Grieve, Mrs. M. *A Modern Herbal*, Jonathan Cape, 1931. Recent editions by Savva Publishing, Adelaide, 1985.

Hoffman, David, *The Holistic Herbal*, Element Books, Shaftesbury, Dorset, 1983.

Lad, Dr Vasant, and Frawley, David, *The Yoga of Herbs*, Lotus Press, Santa Fe, New Mexico, 1986.

Levy, Juliette de Baircli, *The Illustrated Herbal Handbook*, Faber and Faber, 1974.

Lust, John, *The Herb Book*, Bantam Books, New York, 1974.

Lust, John and Tierra, Michael, *The Natural Remedy Bible*, Pocket Books, New York, 1990.

Mabey, Richard (Ed), *The Complete New Herbal*, Penguin Books, 1991.

Messegué, Maurice, *Of Men and Plants*, Weidenfeld and Nicolson, London, 1972.

Nissim, Rina, *Natural Healing in Gynaecology*, Pandora Press, London and New York, 1986.

Pedersen, Mark, *Nutritional Herbology*, Pedersen Publishing, Bountiful, Utah, 1987.

Stuart, Malcolm, *The Encyclopedia of Herbs and Herbalism*, Caxton/ Macdonald & Co., 1989.

Teegarden, Ron, *Chinese Tonic Herbs*, Japan Publications Inc., Tokyo and New York, 1984.

Tierra, Lesley, *The Herbs of Life*, Crossing Press, Freedom, CA 1992.

Tierra, Michael, *The Way of Herbs*, Orenda/Unity Press, 1980.

—*Planetary Herbology*, Lotus Press, Santa Fe, New Mexico, 1988.

Weiss, Rudolf Fritz, *Herbal Medicine*, Beaconsfield Publishers Ltd, Beaconsfield, UK.

Handbooks for identification of herbs

Launert, Edmund, *Edible and Medicinal Plants of Britain and Northern Europe*, Hamlyn, 1981.

Phillips, Roger, *Wild Flowers of Britain*, Pan Books, London, 1981.

—*Wild Flowers of Britain*, Readers Digest, 1981.

Books on Ayurveda and Tibb-Islamic medicine

Chisti, Hakim, G.M. *The Traditional Healer*, Thorsons, 1988.

Khan, Muhammed Salim, *Islamic Medicine*, Routledge and Kegan Paul, London, 1986.

Lad, Dr. Vasant, *Ayurveda: The Science of Self-Healing*, Lotus Press, Santa Fe, New Mexico, 1984.

Books of historical interest, on the history of botanical medicine and man's use of plants

Culpepper's *Complete Herbal and English Physician*, facsimile of 1826 edition, Magna Books, Leicester, 1992.

Edelstein, Ludwig, *Ancient Medicine*, John Hopkins Press, Baltimore, 1967.

Gerard's *Herbal*, Studio Editions, London, 1985.

Griggs, Barbara, *Green Pharmacy*, Jill, Norman and Hobhouse, London, 1981.

Hippocratic Writings, Penguin Books, 1986.

Hutchens, Alma R. *Indian Herbology of North America*, Merco, Windsor, Ontario, Canada, 1969.

Huxley, Anthony, *Green Inheritance*, Gaia Books Ltd, London, 1984.

Manniche, Lise, *An Ancient Egyptian Herbal*, British Museum Publications, 1989.

Phillips, E.D. *Greek Medicine*, Thames and Hudson, London, 1973.

Riddle, John M. *Dioscorides on Pharmacy and Medicine*, University of Texas Press, Austin, 1985.

Tompkins, Peter and Bird, Christopher, *The Secret Life of Plants*, Harper and Row, 1973 and Penguin, 1991.

Periodicals of interest on the modern use of herbs and current scientific research

HerbalGram, Journal of the American Botanical Council and Herb Research Foundation, PO Box 201660, Austin, Texas, USA.

European Journal of Herbal Medicine, National Institute of Medical Herbalists, 9 Palace Gate, Exeter, Devon, UK.

SOURCES OF HERBAL SUPPLIES

Many health-food shops supply good quality dried herbs and some have extended their culinary range to include many more strictly medicinal herbs. In large cities you may find ethnic food shops that carry the traditional herbs of a particular culture.

In the UK Culpepper's shops in the larger towns and cities have a good range of dried herbs, and many companies such as the following supply herbs by mail order and in small quantities.

G. Baldwin & Co., 173 Walworth Road, London SE17 1RW. Tel 071 7035550.

Star Child, 3 The Courtyard, 2–4 High Street, Glastonbury, Somerset BA6 9DU. Tel 0458 834663.

Neal's Yard Remedies, Neal's Yard, Covent Garden, London WC2H 9PD. Tel 071 379 0705.

East-West Herbs, Neal's Yard, Covent Garden, London WC2H 9PD. Tel 071 379 1312.

Napiers Herbalists, 18 Bristol Place, Edinburgh, Tel 031 225 5542.

Vital Force, Hartswood, Marsh Green, Hartfield, E. Sussex TN7 4ET. Tel 0342 282 2312.

Herbs of Grace, 5 Turnpike Road, Red Lodge, Bury St. Edmunds, Suffolk IP28 8JZ. Tel 0638 750140.

Malcolm Simmonds Herbal Supplies, 3 Burton Villas, Hove, Sussex BN3 6FN. Tel 0273 202401.

Self-Heal Herbs, Hayes Corner, South Cheriton, Templecombe, Somerset BA8 OBR. Tel 0963 370300.

Herbal Pillows, Elizabeth Hayes, 2 Station Road, Corsham, Wiltshire SN13 9EX.

The Herbs

*See Materia Medica for details

Agnus castus	*Vitex agnus-castus*
Agrimony	*Agrimonia eupatoria*
Alfalfa	*Medicago sativa*
Allspice	*Syzygium aromaticum* (*Eugenia pimenta*)
Aloe vera* (bitter aloes, medicine plant)	*Aloe vera* (*A. barbadensis*)
Angelica	*Angelica archangelica* (*A. officinalis*)
Anise	*Pimpinella anisum*
Asafoetida	*Ferula assa-foetida*
Ashwaghanda*	*Withania somnifera*
Asparagus	*Asparagus officinalis*
Balm of Gilead (resin)	*Populus* × *Jackii Gileadensis*
Barberry	*Berberis vulgaris*
Basil*	*Ocimum basillicum*
Bay	*Laurus nobilis*
Bayberry*	*Myrica pennsylvanica*
Birch	*Betula* species
Bistort	*Polygonum bistorta*
Blackberry	*Rubus fruticosus*
Black cohosh	*Cimicifuga racemosa*
Black Pepper	*Piper nigrum*
Blue flag iris	*Iris versicolor*
Borage	*Borago officinalis*
Buckwheat	*Polygonum fagopyrum*
Burdock*	*Arctium lappa*

150

Calamus, Sweet* (sweet flag)	*Acorus calamus*
Caraway	*Carum carvi*
Cardamom	*Eletarria cardamomum*
Catnip*	*Nepeta cataria*
Cayenne Pepper*	*Capsicum annuum*
Celery	*Apium graveolens var. dulce*
Chamomile, Roman*	*Chamaemelum nobile*
Chamomile, German*	*Matricaria recutita*
Chaparral* (creosote bush)	*Larrea divaricata*
Chickweed*	*Stellaria media*
Chrysanthemum	*Dendranthema × grandiflorum*
Cinnamon	*Cinnamomum zeylanicum*
Cleavers*	*Galium aparine*
Clove*	*Eugenia caryophyllus*
Coltsfoot*	*Tussilago farfara*
Comfrey*	*Symphytum officinalis*
Coriander	*Coriandrum sativum*
Corn silk (corn-on-the-cob)	*Zea mays*
Couchgrass, twitch	*Triticum repens*
Crampbark* (guelder rose)	*Viburnum opulus*
Cumin*	*Cuminum cyminum*
Cypress	*Cupressus* or *Chaemycyparis* species
Dandelion*	*Taraxacum officinalis*
Dill	*Anethum graveolens*
Dong quai* (Chinese angelica)	*Angelica sinensis*
Echinacea* (coneflower)	*Echinacea angustifolia* and *E. purpurea*
Elderflower* (elderberry)	*Sambucus nigra*
Elecampane	*Inula helenium*
Ephedra	*Ephedra* species
Eucalyptus	*Eucalyptus globulus*
Evening primrose	*Oenothera* species
Eyebright	*Euphrasia officinalis*
False unicorn	*Helonius bullata* (*H. dioica*)
Fennel*	*Foeniculum vulgare*
Fenugreek	*Trigonella foenum-graecum*
Feverfew	*Tanacetum parthenium*
Flax, linseed	*Linum usitatissimum*
Garlic*	*Allium sativum*
Gentian, yellow	*Gentiana lutea* (*G. officinalis*)
Ginger*	*Zingiber officinalis*
Ginseng*	*Panax ginseng*
Ginseng, American*	*Panax quinquefolium*

Golden seal*	*Hydrastis canadensis*
Gotu Kola* (Indian pennywort)	*Hydrocotle (Centella asiatica)*
Ground ivy	*Glechoma hederacea*
Hawthorn*	*Crataegus oxycantha (C. laevigata)*
Heather	*Erica or Colluna species*
Heartsease (pansy)	*Viola tricolor; V. × wittrockiana*
Hibiscus	*Hibiscus rosa-sinensis*
Hollyhock	*Alcea rosea*
Honeysuckle	*Lonicera saponica*
Hop*	*Humulus lupulus*
Horseradish	*Amoracia rusticana*
Horsetail* (marestail)	*Equisetum arvense*
Hyssop*	*Hyssopus officinalis*
Iceland moss	*Cetraria islandica*
Irish moss	*Chondrus crispus*
Jujube, Indian	*Zizyphus mauritanica*
Juniper*	*Juniperus communis*
Kelp* (bladderwrack)	*Fucus vesiculosis*
Kudzu vine	*Pueraria lobata*
Lady's mantle	*Alchemilla vulgaris (A. xanthochlora)*
Lavender	*Lavandula angustifolia (L. officinalis)*
Lemon balm*	*Melissa officinalis*
Lemongrass	*Cymbopogon citratus*
Licorice*	*Glycyrrhiza glabra*
Lime tree	*Tilia species*
Lobelia, Indian tobacco*	*Lobelia inflata*
Lungwort	*Pulmonaria officinalis*
Marjoram	*Origanum majorana*
Marigold* (calendula)	*Calendula officinalis*
Marshmallow*	*Althaea officinalis*
Mint *see* peppermint	
Mistletoe	*Viscum album*
Meadowsweet*	*Filipendula ulmaria*
Motherwort	*Leonurus cardiaca*
Mullein*	*Verbascum thapsus*
Mung bean	*Vigna radiata*
Myrrh	*Commifera myrrha*
Nasturtium	*Nasturtium officinalis*
Nettle*	*Urtica urens*
Nutmeg	*Myristica fragrans*
Oak	*Quercus species*
Oats	*Avena sativa*

Oregon grape*	*Mahonia aquifolium*
Parsley*	*Petroselinum crispum*
Passionflower, wild	*Passiflora incarnata*
Peony	*Paeonia alba*
Peppermint, spearmint,*	*Mentha piperita, M. spicata,*
horsemint and pennyroyal	*M. arvensis* and *M. pulegium*
Plantain,* psyllium seeds	*Plantago major, P. indica*
Periwinkle	*Vinca major*
Pleurisy root	*Asclepias tuberosa*
Poke root	*Phytolacca americana*
Poplar bark	*Populus balsamifera, P. nigra.*
	P. tremuloides
Raspberry*	*Rubus idaeus*
Red clover*	*Trifolium pratense*
Rose geranium	*Pelargonium graveolens*
Rosemary*	*Rosmarinus officinalis*
Sage*	*Salvia officinalis*
Sarsaparilla	*Smilax glauca, ornata*
Sassafras*	*Sassafras albidum*
Saw palmetto	*Serenoa serrulata*
Sandalwood	*Santalum album*
Self heal	*Prunella vulgaris*
Senna	*Cassia acutifolia*
Sesame seeds	*Sesamum indicum*
Shepherd's purse (pennycress)	*Capsella bursa-pastoris*
Skullcap*	*Scutellaria lateriflora*
Slippery elm*	*Ulmus rubra*
Solomon's seal	*Polygonatum odoratum*
Spikenard	*Nardostachys grandiflora*
Squaw vine (partridge berry)	*Mitchella repens*
St John's wort	*Hypericum perforatum*
Thyme*	*Thymus vulgaris*
Ti-tree	*Leptospermum* species
Turkey rhubarb	*Rheum palmatum*
Turmeric*	*Curcuma longa*
Uva-ursi (bearberry)	*Arctostaphylos uva-ursi*
Valerian*	*Valeriana officinalis*
Vervain	*Verbena officinalis*
Violet	*Viola odorata*
Walnut	*Juglans* species
White oak*	*Quercus alba*
White bark pine*	*Pinus albicaulis* (strobus)
White willow*	*Salix alba*
Wild strawberry	*Fragaria vesca*

Wild yam* (Chinese yam)	*Dioscorea villosa, D. batatus*
Willow bark	*Salix alba, S. nigra*
Wintergreen	*Gaultheria procumbens*
Witch hazel	*Hamamelis species*
Wood betony	*Stachys officinalis*
Woundwort	*Stachys sylvatica*
Yarrow*	*Achillea millefolium*
Yellow dock	*Rumex crispus*

Glossary

Adaptogen: agent that enables the body to deal with and recover from stress and disease.

Allopathic medicine: 'orthodox' medicine, in which drugs are used to oppose and alleviate disease.

Analgesic: pain relieving.

Anodyne: pain relieving.

Antibiotic: combats infection.

Anti-inflammatory: reduces swelling, sheet and pain due to irritation, infection or injury.

Antipyretic: reduces fever.

Antiseptic: controls infection and helps prevent tissue degeneration.

Antispasmodic: relieves cramp.

Astringent: contracts, tightens and binds tissues.

Calcination: process of refining by roasting or burning.

Carminative: expels gas trapped in intestines, improves digestion.

Contraindication: any factor that makes it unwise to pursue a certain line of treatment.

Demulcent: soothing agent that protects mucous membranes and relieves irritation.

Detoxicant: eliminates poisons.

Diaphoretic: causes increase in perspiration and release of waste via the skin.

Distillation: process of extracting essence of plants by heating to vapour, condensing by cooling, and re-collecting liquid.

Diuretic: increases urine and excretion.

Emmenagogue: promotes and regularizes menstrual flow.

Expectorant: removes excess mucous from bronchial tubes.

Filtration: process to filter out impurities.

Haemostatic: arrests bleeding/haemorrhage.

Homoeostasis: physiological process by which the systems of the body are maintained naturally at equilibrium.

Hypertension: high blood pressure.

Laxative: aids bowel evacuation.

Leucorrhoea: whitish or yellowish vaginal discharge.

Mucilage: thick aqueous solution used as a lubricant.

Nervine: reduces nervous disorders.

Oedema: excessive accumulation of fluid in the body.

Pathogen: any agent that causes disease, for example bacteria.

Purgative: aids bowel evacuation.

Sepsis: putrefactive destruction of tissues by disease-causing bacteria or their toxins.

Stasis: stagnation or cessation of flow.

Stimulant: increases one or more of the metabolic processes, such as blood circulation, perspiration, adrenalin secretion.

Stomachic: relieves gastric disorders. Tones stomach.

Sublimation: process of converting from solid state to vapour by heat and allowing to solidify again.

Sudorific: increases perspiration.

Tachycardia: increase in heart rate above normal.

Vulnerary: arrests bleeding in wounds and prevents tissue degeneration.

Index